CONVERSATIONS
ON THE
E D G E

Praise for *Conversations on the Edge*

"In an era when bioethics is increasingly defined by regulation-writing, outcomes assessment, and the exercise of authority, we get Zaner's *Conversations on the Edge*, a now old-fashioned but nonetheless revered immersion in the nitty-gritty of medical morality, complete with the stench of wounds, the tightening grip of anguish, and the fusion of doubt and hope. Bless him!"

> —John Z. Sadler, M.D., professor and director, Undergraduate
> Medical Education, Department of Psychiatry, The University
> of Texas Southwestern Medical Center at Dallas

"These moving conversations and reflections place the reader squarely at the bedside, where ethical decision making is deeply situated in the agonizing dilemmas confronted by the sick. In providing extraordinary insights into the experience of patients, family members, and those involved in their care, Zaner's book is an invaluable resource for all who are interested in clinical ethics."

> —S. Kay Toombs, author of *The Meaning of Illness* and emeritus
> associate professor of philosophy, Baylor University

"Ethical dilemmas are human problems; personal struggles over finding the right thing to do. When ethicists step in to help, these problems reverberate within them as persons also. We read a lot about the ethical issues, but it takes someone of Richard Zaner's extraordinary sensitivity and superb observational skills to take us into his thoughts and inner debates to show us the personal magnitude of ethics for all the participants. This book adds a vital dimension to the study of bioethics."

> —Eric J. Cassell, M.D., M.A.C.P, clinical professor of public health,
> Weill Medical College of Cornell University

"Zaner has fearlessly reconceptualized ethics practice as a reflexive relatedness to others, achieved and enacted through narrative means, that opens self and others to truth. This book is a stunning accomplishment of daring, transformative, Jamesian respect for freedom."

> —Rita Charon, professor of clinical medicine and director of the
> Program in Narrative Medicine, Columbia University

CONVERSATIONS
ON THE
EDGE

Narratives of Ethics and Illness

Richard M. Zaner

Georgetown University Press/Washington, D.C.

Georgetown University Press, Washington, D.C.
© 2004 by Georgetown University Press. All rights reserved.
Printed in the United States of America

10 9 8 7 6 5 4 3 2 1   2004

This book is printed on acid-free recycled paper meeting the
requirements of the American National Standard for Perma-
nence in Paper for Printed Library Materials.

Library of Congress Cataloging-in-Publication Data

Zaner, Richard M.
    Conversations on the edge : narratives of ethics and illness
/ Richard M. Zaner
            p.   cm.
Includes bibliographical references.
    ISBN 0-87840-348-5 (alk. paper)
1. Medical ethics—Case studies.   2. Sick—Psychology.
3. Physician and patient.   I. Title.
    R724.Z355 2004
    174.2—dc22   2003019459

This is for Mark Bliton and Stuart Finder, colleagues and friends, for those astonishing, enriching years together.

And, for my children, Melora and Andrew, who glow with such incredible promise.

You've made my life a wondrous journey.

Contents

Preface   xi

1. Quiet Rooms for Troubled Voices   1
2. When You're Dead Anyway, What's to Live For?   17
3. Hope against Hope   39
4. Don't Let Me Forget to Remember   69
5. Broader's Hill   89
6. The Cruel Clarity of It All   111

Acknowledgments   143
Notes   147

Preface

> Human language is like a cracked kettle on which we
> beat out tunes for bears to dance to, when all the
> time we are longing to move the stars to pity.
> —Gustave Flaubert

I am well aware that there is considerable variety in these writings.
It is also true that I find myself mixing different styles within a single
story.

In part, this is by design. In another way, though, it is not in the
least that I had a plan worked out in advance of the actual writing and
had merely to stretch the stories onto some sort of Procrustean bed.
I should also make it clear that I do not, not yet at least, fully understand just what this means—neither for myself nor for the craft of
writing. I did not deliberately set out to confound anyone; nor in
some idle moment did I decide to wear the guise of a really clever
guy, trying my hand first at this, then dancing with quick cunning
into another of a menu of available genres. I wanted, rather, to be as
honest as I could to the situations that initially gave rise to these stories, my involvement in each of them, to listen internally and
intensely—but now with much more focused reflection and with the
utmost care—to what each of the original encounters seemed to be
about, to what each seemed bent on having told, as well as what my
experiences as involved helped me to understand and, I hope, say in
writing. It is true that I still find myself learning from the writing of
these stories far more and far deeper than I would have ever thought
possible before.

Several of these writings are quite new and assumed a form very
different from anything I have written before. Several others are
modified from lectures I delivered, and I had it in mind to try and
keep something of the spontaneity of the original lectures. Still others are complete rewrites of stories I have told earlier, rewritten

because I have long been dissatisfied with the way I first wrote them—as they just did not allow much of the sense and passion of the original to come through the words I used then. Now, I have tried to be more faithful to the original occasions—hopefully in the sense James Agee may have had in mind in that remarkable book, *Let Us Now Praise Famous Men*, he and Walker Evans published together with Evans's stunning photographs:

> For in the immediate world, everything is to be discerned, for him who can discern it, and centrally and simply, without either dissection into science, or digestion into art, but with the whole of consciousness, seeking to perceive it as it stands: so that the aspect of a street in sunlight can roar in the heart of itself as a symphony, perhaps as no symphony can: and all of consciousness is shifted from the imagined, the revisive, to the effort to perceive simply the cruel radiance of what is. [1]

Like Agee, I wanted to do nothing more than let these things and people be, whatever they are and in whatever way they might (want to) be, with neither dissection nor digestion. I hope to make it very clear that I believe Agee is right, and though I realize how hard it is to stand in that "cruel radiance," I think I understand why that is so important as regards the situations whose various circumstances and people play out in these stories—and to which I now return.

Two of them were previously published in forms very different from what is found here. The story of Tom and his mother—"When You're Dead, What's to Live For?"—was, in a much shorter version, included in my first book of stories, *Troubled Voices*. [2] The story about my mother's final moments—"The Cruel Clarity of It All"— first appeared as part of a chapter in my earlier book, *Ethics and the Clinical Encounter*, [3] but I identified neither myself nor my mother, and many details vital to the story presented here were not in the earlier version. I retell it now for many reasons, mainly having to do with my dogged efforts to get it right, so I could work through my guilt and make my peace with those troubled and still troubling events.

"Don't Let Me Forget to Remember" first appeared as the main part of a grand rounds lecture for the Section of Surgery at Vanderbilt University Medical Center, about a year after the events related in it. I then used it as a basis for several other lectures for different groups, trying each time to get right what I had experienced. "Hope against Hope" was delivered as a plenary address to the European Society for Philosophy of Medicine and Health Care at its 1999 meeting in Linköping, Sweden. Titled "Power and Hope in the Clinical Encounter: A Meditation on Vulnerability," it was later published in the Society's journal.[4] That lecture was in turn based on an earlier invited article, "Encountering the Other," published in an anthology.[5] The chapter I call "Quiet Rooms for Troubled Voices" was first presented as the Inaugural Christine Martin Lecture at the University of Melbourne, Australia.[6] Before now, it, "Don't Let Me Forget to Remember," and "Broader's Hill" have never been published in any form.

"Broader's Hill" is without doubt the most difficult and oddest piece I have ever written. I think the present version is the most coherent of the many that preceded it, though it may be the easiest to get through. Not that I have not gone over it—many, many times—nor that I have not edited and reedited. I have done all that, but I have been unable to make it come out much differently. Frankly, I continue to be utterly taken by that encounter, and in its original form it attempted to capture the original experience as it happened, as much as possible. It was a particularly difficult ethics consult, one that brought out certain thematic issues for me about many such encounters and about writing. I hope the present version does justice to what that encounter prompted.

It is clear that I have been thinking and fretting over some of the same themes for a long time. I think, however, that anyone familiar with my earlier writings, the stories especially, will find a good deal that is new here. I know I have, even while I also recognize that the centering themes persist through most of what I have written since my first published essay in 1961.

After many years in the world of medicine and health care, the last twenty plus mainly in clinical and research settings, I have come to think that it is not so much autonomy that lies at the basis of our lives as moral creatures, nor does it constitute the basic moral fact of our lives. It is rather, to put it one way, the responsibility that each of us bears to *respect* the autonomy, the *self* and the *life and humanity* of the other, the one who is profoundly vulnerable thanks to illness, injury, or the social and personal devastations of genetic disease—at whatever stage or condition of life that self or person may be and in appreciation of all its significant and subtle implications.

What I encountered in each of the stories in this book is just how deeply we are each shaped by our multiple connections with other people—from the always mysterious stirrings that subtly announce to a woman that her pregnancy is under way, and where chance rules like nothing else,[7] to the more obvious movements of a fetus almost ready to enter the world and on to those awesome times when death is clear, present, and commanding. Most of us may be quite surprised when we find ourselves stunned, in tears, gripped by grief we yet only barely recognize and understand, or how we can be shaken by what we inarticulately but powerfully feel when faced with the loss of someone intimate and dear, at whatever age it may be. I certainly was when I was with my dying mother as I sat and watched those awesome monitors slowly sink and flatten, as I think Tom and his mother were shocked by the finality portended in his rejection of dialysis in the second story included here. Eventually, in a stunning moment, he and his mother came to realize that, yes, Tom would certainly die if he persisted in his stated "choice" to refuse dialysis. I was certainly astounded in my meetings with them, too, as I am sure were the parents of the premature twins in my first story, by the very presence and depth of their connection with those tiny babies, neither of whom had managed to survive more than a few days and who yet exercised such power over their thoughts and dreams.

As I found myself working and writing my way through these situations, reflecting on them time and again, I found I was often dwelling on the same issues, the same questions. Why is it that in the face of grievous illness, injury, or the devastation of genetic accidents, people more often than not manifest connections with others so intense that surprise marks the experience quite as much as dismay or grief? What are those links or bonds: between Tom and his mother, Jim and Sue and their twins, and to myself as well? Or, how was it that Mrs. Oland, in "Hope against Hope," so clearly understood what her husband was going through even as she was dying and pretty much out of it—while he was so deeply in the throes of profound sadness and guilt? Or that bright, intelligent mother facing her son's imminent death, in "Broader's Hill," just knowing, feeling he was still alive and "there," despite the odds and the neurologist's firm and contrary words: did her sense, and the decisions that stemmed from it, effectively only prolong her son's inevitable death? How could she think that her son was after all really alive in that husk of remaining body? Or my standing there in the intensive care unit, watching the monitors record the last moments of my mother's life, and how could I still, despite everything, feel the nagging twinges of guilt? Did my mother come finally to the point where she had to take things into her own hands, there being no Kevorkian about to help? If you had been there—at Tom's bedside with his mother right there, with those tiny twins and Jim and Sue right there, with Mr. Oland, or with that young mother and her remaining son—would you have known what was going on and what ought to be done? Not even my own facing myself in the midst of that wild talk at the neurobiology conference escapes such questions, for the embedded fear I found in myself—despite or because of my knowing better?—and in others gives ample and poignant evidence about how Alzheimer's and other neurologically debilitating diseases give us such inward shudders. What is this but the dread of finding ourselves so demented as no longer to know ourselves or recognize our own faces in the mirror, or the faces of those we hold most dear? Or, on the other side of this, to be witness to the loss of self when we are no longer recognized by someone we love, who is now in the grip of a disease that strips self from its embodiment even while the body remains? What are these connections with others all about? And how can we understand when such situations happen to us?

Roger Rosenblatt noted, in a *Time* magazine editorial, that each of us is inevitably caught up in such challenges—which, he tells us, is why we are always telling stories to one another:

> So much of living is made of storytelling that one might con-
> clude that it is what we were meant to do—to tell one another
> stories, fact or fiction, as a way of keeping afloat. . . . We have the
> story of others to tell, or of ourselves, or of the species—some
> monumentally elusive tale we are always trying to get right.[8]

Nor is getting that monumentally elusive tale right at all easy, certainly not for me. In these and other writings, I am constantly brought up against those riddles that beleaguer, pester, and yet somehow define everything we do and what we ultimately are.

It is not easy to talk or write honestly about such situations; it is all the more awkward and difficult to do so when someone intimate to you is faced with the extreme situation: someone close and dear is dying, or being born, or becoming increasingly demented. It is for most of us next to impossible when the person in question is oneself. Faced with such situations, Ronald Blythe's terse comment about Tolstoy's *The Death of Ivan Ilych* comes to mind: that like Ivan Ilych, each of us knows intimately the "plight of a man who has a coldly adequate language for dealing with another's death but who remains incoherent when it comes to his own."[9] Except that, for a lot of us, not even that coldly adequate language is always ready to hand, nor does it give sense and substance to our experience even when we do find it.

So if at times my language, as Flaubert said, seems only "like a cracked kettle" on which I manage merely to "beat out tunes for

bears to dance to," I hope you will keep in mind that I really am trying to get each story right, hoping "to move the stars to pity."

Finally, I must note here that I have changed everything that
might otherwise be used to identify any of the people involved in the
encounters narrated in these pages, except myself.

CONVERSATIONS
ON THE
E D G E

Narratives of Ethics and Illness

1

Quiet Rooms for Troubled Voices

Years ago, not long after the time I first became a somewhat regular, if also odd, presence in our newborn intensive care unit, or NICU, one of the attending physicians in the unit, Dr. Peter Shannon, had asked a nurse, Rebecca Warren, to ask me to meet with the parents of twins, both born recently very prematurely, and both currently in the unit.[1]

Rebecca told me the babies were "preemies" and that one of them, it seemed as certain as these things can be—not often very certain at all—would surely not make it. The other baby, she said, though with serious complications, still might survive. If it did, like so many of these extremely premature infants, though, it would most likely have more or less severe neurological problems. It was just not possible to predict these things well.

I forget what the twins' problems were, though they were doubtless not untypical of many premature infants: hypoxia and asphyxia resulting in abnormal breathing requiring ventilation at unusually high settings that could cause still other problems, such as blindness: too much oxygen, blindness; too little, brain damage or death. It was also likely that the babies had suffered some form of brain insult due to hemorrhage, which could result in cerebral palsy or other brain damage. There was, also, persistent hypotension, damage to the delicate lung tissue (pneumothoraces), with tubes stuck into the chest to drain accumulating fluids, and other problems that challenge even the most competent and caring neonatologist.

But what Rebecca had begun to tell me about these twins—problems as unwanted as they are common—is not the story and in fact was not what prompted a request from the attending physician that I talk with the babies' parents and, perhaps later, members of the NICU as well.

"We're really concerned, about these parents," Rebecca said, "especially the father."

"Oh? Why?"—it was the only thing I could say at the time and in the face of her worried expression.

This situation occurred very early in my work in the unit, in fact quite early in my unnerving transformation from a professor of philosophy to practicing clinician—someone trying very hard to learn how to identify issues, clarify options, get people to talk in order to help them, those who must make at times harsh decisions in the face of real or imagined ethical problems, dilemmas, even the sort of enigma where nobody knows more than that there is something deeply troubling and that it must somehow still be worked through—and when none of this is on some printed page, or like correct answers at the back of a textbook.

"Well," she explained to my inexperienced ear, "he doesn't talk. . . ."

"What do you mean, 'Doesn't talk'?" I was a bit impatient, I admit.

"Give me a chance," she said, and went on to explain how, when Dr. Shannon went to talk with the parents about the one twin—the one who would likely not make it—the father just stood there, stiff and expressionless, neither nodding his head nor showing the slightest glint of understanding. When he repeated what he had to tell the parents and went on to explain that there was some hope the second twin might do all right, still, not a whisper of response. "It was like he hadn't heard a thing," was Dr. Shannon's report.

"What about the mother?" I wondered. "You didn't mention her. Is she there when the attending talks to her husband? Does the doctor talk to her, too?"

"Oh, sure," Rebecca quickly responded.

"How does she respond?" I asked. "How is she taking it?"

"Well, to tell the truth, she seems just devastated," Rebecca said, and went on: "She breaks into tears at the first word. She just seems totally out of it; like she knows and doesn't want to know and can't stand to know, but knows she has to know, and then turns to her husband. But, well, he's like made of stone. And, you know, they're both so young!"

"Young? How young?"

She told me that both parents were in their early twenties; the father was twenty-five and the mom twenty-three. "This is their first pregnancy," she said, "and both of them seem really well educated; when the babies were first brought in, at least he said something then, and he seemed well spoken."

Which made me wonder aloud, "'Brought in,' you said. Where were the twins born?" I was wondering whether something untoward might have occurred either at the other hospital during delivery or during transport.

Rebecca pointed out that the babies were "outliers" transported to our NICU by Angel II, our unit's fully equipped mobile NICU, and that the twins' problems were, so far as the doctors could tell, because of their premature birth, not due to problems during delivery or transport or to inappropriate care at the other hospital.

"Do you know what the father does, where he works?" I asked after a moment to think about what she'd told me thus far. "Does the mother work, too?"

"Yeah, I think they both work. He's got some sort of executive-type job with some big company locally. He wears a suit and tie every time I see him. She, I think, does something similar and also dresses really nice. I'm not really sure, but they both seem well educated, college types."

"What do you think his silence means?" I asked, getting back on track a bit.

That she didn't give a direct answer to the question, I was later to learn, itself harbored serious, if somewhat hidden meaning. Now, though, I noted only that she said, "It just isn't normal, not when the attending keeps trying to get him and his wife to decide about the first twin. Treatments," she emphasized, "are just not doing any good, and Dr. Shannon is just trying to make sure they understand that, well, that maybe now the time has come to, well, to recognize that nothing seems to help. . . ."

She herself clearly had real difficulty saying this, so, without giving it much thought, I blundered out with, "You mean that it's time to discontinue treatments, to let the baby die?" I had already been involved in several similar situations, so, though I was somewhat brusque, at least I had the presence of mind to know that the question had to be asked. I did, though, say it softly, quietly.

Anyway, she acknowledged the point and repeated that she, Dr. Shannon, and others on the care team were worried about this father: why was he so rigid, so restrained? "He's just setting himself up for some hard times, you know?" she emphasized. Silence like his just wasn't what you'd expect, wasn't what was most often heard from practically any parent when it became clear that treatments were only prolonging the inevitable, that death is near and must be acknowledged.

Many parents, maybe most, she pointed out, most often insisted that doctors keep on treating their baby, keep doing everything possible even when, truth be told, "everything" had already been done; that demand or request, I was quickly learning, was among the most common I would hear in such situations. Rebecca knew, she said, that it takes time for parents to come to the point where they eventually understand, where they can accept and then come to a decision with the unit team about the inevitable, the futility of continuing to treat their baby.

This father, however, had been told many times already, and every time he kept his stony, stubborn silence. Rebecca didn't know whether the father talked with his wife—or she to him—about this, but when they were together with nurses or doctors, she invariably looked to him for decisions, or so it seemed. But he was restrained, wordless, closed in, even, seemingly, unaffected. He did not seem to hear: no tears, words, gestures, nothing—and *that* was what worried them, that almost tangible, even cagey reserve.

So, I was asked to talk with the parents, although at the time I hardly knew what I should say, nor had I yet understood that it was better for me to listen than to talk, far more to help get their thoughts identified and addressed than any I had. This was one of the encounters that really helped bring that home to me.

When I went into the room that had been set aside for our meeting, they were sitting there just like Rebecca had reported. She was quietly weeping; his reserve was palpable. Perhaps because of Rebecca's description, the silence seemed menacing. He glared at me when I came in, as if daring me to say something.

I felt as though I were on the edge of a precipice: one wrong word and all would be lost, things would cave in like mud—with me left unclear whether or how I might be somehow to blame. I even wondered whether I should just say "hi" and leave: I could say I made a mistake, got into the wrong room, and just take off.

But I couldn't. Instead, I searched for words to console, reassure, commiserate, unsure until the last moment what could possibly be the right words at a time like this, or whether I could talk at all.

But I did. First off, I introduced myself. For reasons I can't fathom, the words that came out sounded bizarre to me, and I'm sure to them. I hadn't introduced myself that way ever before. First my name, then I blurted out, "I'm a philosopher, the doctors and nurses in the NICU have asked me to talk with you."

But before I could complete the sentence, he—let me call him Jim, his wife Sue—suddenly got an incredulous look on his face, one of utter disbelief. Sue stopped weeping, abruptly glanced up at me with an obviously perplexed, if still weepy look. I just knew that I'd blown it.

"A philosopher?" Jim demanded, his admirable candor providing all the inflection he needed. "What in the world is a philosopher doing here?" A not unreasonable question, I thought and said so, wondering what, indeed, I *was* doing there.

Striving to recover from losing any more ground, I quickly tried to say what sort of thing I did in the NICU and in the hospital. And just then it hit me: what *do* I do? Moreover, what is "a philosopher" doing in such a place? But never mind that—*really*, never mind what I went on to say to Jim and Sue. Although that's a continuing issue for anyone who decides to get involved in clinical settings, it was not an issue for them, as quickly became clear.

As I now think about it, two things struck me right off about the situation. First, neither of them seemed in the least interested in what I then fumbled about trying to say. Despite Jim's explosive "What the hell . . . ?" and Sue's open-mouthed gape, that was obviously simply not something they were much concerned about. Second, and even more striking for me, was that, as I went on talking about what I do—reaching for each subsequent word as the previous one somehow slipped out—Jim was becoming increasingly animated.

Shortly, he erupted. "Never mind all that. Why," he bluntly asked, "are you here now?" And with, again, exemplary frankness, he pointedly demanded, eyes narrowing in that knowing way, full of suspicion: "Has someone been acting unethically?"

Ah, the bane of my life: for the first couple of years in this practice, every time I introduced myself, it seemed, someone invariably thought that, since I was "in ethics," it was obvious that somebody had been *un*ethical; otherwise, why else would someone like me be on the scene? And I, taken to be the local "ethics cop," was there to catch 'em out and put 'em away! Curious, and not a little frustrating, how being seen as "police"—even if merely from "ethics"—puts such a damper on conversation.

In any event, Jim seemed a bit embarrassed by his outburst and quietly listened as I told them that, no, nobody to my knowledge had done anything wrong, nor was that why I was there, not at all. Rather, and I went on to explain how many of the medical and nursing staff had been concerned about them, him in particular, how his reticence and stony silences were so disturbing and that perhaps he'd like to talk about that, about what the doctors and nurses had been telling them about their babies.

Did he, did she, did they understand what had been going on? Had he and his wife been listening, had they heard what they were told? Did they understand specifically what they were being asked to recognize, to accept, to agree to, to decide on, eventually to live with?

And, again, with surprising openness and before I could finish my thought, he drove straight to the point: *of course*, he understood, and so did Sue—she nodded vigorously, her hands never quite still, tears still glistening in her eye and on her cheek, despite the slightly amused look she had as I stumbled trying to tell them what a "philosopher," or at least this one, does in the hospital.

Jim affirmed the obvious: they knew perfectly well that the first twin was going to die. I noted that he used the awful words few can use—dying, death—especially in these situations. Despite every effort to stabilize, correct, or only ameliorate the baby's condition (yes, he and she were "educated," enough at least to use some pretty sophisticated language, and with remarkably correct grammar), the first twin was surely dying and the second's condition did not bode at all well.

"Yes, I know," Jim said, now talking more rapidly, "both of us know full well that our babies aren't doing at all well, that Seth"— he's the first twin, a boy—"is going to die, and that Beth"—the second, a girl—"will likely also not make it, certainly not without serious neurological damage, but we just don't think it is fair to her, to Beth, to force her to live that kind of life. But with Seth, we know that there's nothing more that can be done; it's only a question of time before he dies, probably in the next couple of days, if not before," and he slowly grew quiet, as if wearied by his outburst of words and the burden of what was, for him, so clearly and deeply agonizing.

"How come you haven't told the doctors, then?" I wondered, admittedly somewhat mystified. Why was he so vocal *with me? Does being a philosopher do that to people?*

Those musings to the side, Jim came right to the point: "You think we *haven't* told them? Of *course*, we have!" But then he seemed to back off, to hesitate, then seemed on the verge of another torrent of words that, however, didn't happen. He stopped talking; he withdrew into himself, into that dark, besetting place where he had been secluded for so many weeks.

When I pointed out how restrained, at times even hostile, he at least appeared to be, with evident effort he crawled back out again, his voice now meditative, profoundly, inescapably sad.

He began again to talk. He said that, though it was unplanned, they joyfully welcomed the pregnancy, especially how eagerly they had looked forward to having twins. The idea of twins had somehow piqued their fancy. When Sue went into premature labor (at about twenty-five weeks gestational age), thus, it was not entirely unexpected. Still, they rushed to the local hospital, but her labor couldn't be stopped and suddenly, before anything could be done, she gave birth to the twins. They were then promptly brought to our NICU. Things seemed to go well for a while, but gradually, and with agonizing and seemingly inexorable certainty, it became very clear that both of the babies were suffering with terribly difficult problems. And then, of course, the really bad news had come.

Well, he continued, late one evening while in their motel room, he and Sue were not so much watching as just staring at the television, when it began to dawn on them that what they were watching sounded very much like what they were going through. It was that night back in the mid-1980s when on his regular show, *Nightline*, Ted Koppel interviewed the parents of "Baby Jane Doe"—the severely premature baby girl in Long Island afflicted with microcephaly and spina bifida. Because of the pathologically tiny head and enlarged brain ventricles, not only did brain damage and severe mental retardation seem all but certain, but so, too, would the baby be physically disabled, thanks to the lesion on her spinal column, and would thus face many years of surgeries, medicines, crutches, braces, the lot. Her parents had not wanted the spinal lesion closed, had not wanted to force their baby to live, had decided to do nothing. And, though they were appalled by their own decision, they continued to feel it was the only thing to do, that it was "right," and that they would be supported by their church. Catholics, they were, in fact, supported by their priest and even the bishop, as well as the physician and the hospital. All agreed. Then, they found themselves being sued by an attorney who lived hundreds of miles away, with the intent of forcing surgical closure of the lesion on the premise that all life, no matter how desperate or damaged, is sacred and that everything must be done to preserve it.

With one side winning, then another, the case had been appealed through every level of court in the state of New York and eventually wound up in the New York Supreme Court, where the judges rejected the initial suit and informed the attorney who had brought the original suit that he had no legal standing in the first place. The case was then appealed to the United States Supreme Court, which upheld the parents' refusal to allow access to their baby's medical records. Thus, it was ripe subject matter for television as well.

Jim had reacted passionately to the images of that father testifying in one court after another, at one point being shown with a brown paper bag over his head—to protect, he said to Mr. Koppel on national television, the pitifully little that was still left of his privacy. Jim saw himself, his wife, their family, everyone they cared about, being held up to public ridicule. He had become vehement, Sue said, vowing that he would never put his family through such a circus.

But how could anybody prevent that, especially in such a media-hyped time as ours? Jim had somehow gotten the idea into his head that, if he could just keep his silence, if he said nothing at all whenever anyone asked him what he wanted done, then whatever "decision" was eventually made would be, not his, but the doctors'! Then, if anybody tried to put them on public display by suing them, well, he would say, the decision wasn't his, he had no part of it; it was the doctors who did it! Then, he could protect his family from the horrendous experience of being publicly exposed, laid bare by, and in, the media.

All of which, he now obviously recognized, did not so much constitute reasons as were expressions of his own apprehensions over his babies. At this point, it was relatively easy to bring things to some closure. Jim was, after all, becoming rather talkative and was clearly eager to discuss matters with me and, at my urging, with the staff. A meeting was arranged with all those involved present—for apologies, Jim insisted, but also for fuller understanding and especially for much-needed acknowledgments and decisions. Actions were agreed to: what had been called "life supports," but were seen now as "death prolongers," were removed, and Seth was allowed to die. And, despite all their suffering, Jim and Sue were able to accept that Beth's condition was also hopeless. With her death, the terrible issues in this case were brought to a close—even if not a happy one for any of those directly involved.

"Any problem," Hans Jonas, a teacher of mine many years ago, once remarked, "is essentially the collision between a comprehensive view (be it hypothesis or belief) and a particular fact which will not fit." So what we're after when faced with a "problem," so that we can then understand and know what to reckon with, is getting clear about some "collision." The more serious the problem, the more the collision augurs a disaster reaching right down to our inmost lives, trying as best we can to find some constancy between that and our own comprehensive view of things.

But do we ever know what our own beliefs truly are, what the big picture is, much less something so grand as our comprehensive view of the world? From what I've seen, most people have neither thought much about the matter, nor do they really want to do that. That's one of the reasons why situations involving serious illness or injury provoke such passion and uncertainty combined with the sense that people must nevertheless come to a decision. We're supposed to make choices when what we have to base them on is unclear, confusing, ambiguous, unsure.

Which today seems to me just what Jim and Sue were trying to tell the doctors, nurses, and me as their babies were dying. In fact, that's pretty much what I went through when my own mother was dying before my very eyes.[2] What happened to *her*? *Where did she go?* And *why?* I was baffled and now wondered whether such questions were what Rebecca and Dr. Shannon also went through? Even more, did Jim and Sue go through it not once, but twice, with each of their babies?

As you might suspect, there seems much more to the story. If we're always trying to tell our story, what is mine? What happened to Jim and Sue seems but a harbinger of something else.

A character in one of Barry Lopez's lovely fables tells two young ones, Crow and Weasel, during their passage into adulthood that stories "take care of people." Stories are thus gifts, ways we have of helping each other get through bad times. For the same reason, we have to learn to give away our stories when they seem needed by someone else. "Sometimes a person needs a story more than food to stay alive. That is why we put these stories in each other's memory." This, too, is one of the ways we have to help people care for themselves: stories form the grist of our connections with other people.[3]

My gift to Jim and Sue was listening; their gift to me was their story, the one they slowly understood took care of them when they desperately needed to be cared for. And, because of that I took on the burden of telling their story, an obligation from their gift to me. I have now fulfilled some part, at least, of that obligation by making it available now, here, to whoever might chance to read it.

Thinking about this, the writing and rewriting of it especially, I begin to understand, too, just how much Jim and Sue needed to tell their story. Or, at least, to tell *a* story, since you may never be all that certain, I suppose, just which one will or even needs to come out. Sometimes, in fact, it takes a lot of telling before you get it right.

What is this all about? What is so puzzling for me is not just telling and listening, giving and receiving, to each other—magic of their own sort. It's also that such tales and anecdotes are, when heard, so powerful. How they can amaze and move us. Stories also harbor the powerful tug of "obligation" and "responsibility." If I tell a story, I sense that I have a responsibility, among other things, to get it right, to make sense, to be clear, as well as to tell my tale in an interesting way. I also have a responsibility to be faithful to what my story is about. And, if I listen, I bear the responsibility to really listen, not just pretend, and, as listener, to give back to the teller, even though it may be that this giving back is most often a giving to others different from those whose story it was.

Sue told me at one point that she was not only deeply sad at what happened to her babies, but also that she felt "for all the world like I did something to cause it, you know?" Jim, too, said he couldn't quite "get beyond that, that maybe I did something to cause it all." What should I make of that? It seems obvious enough that neither of them "did" anything to "cause it," and they could even agree with that. Yet they felt differently from what on the other hand they knew full well. Why is that?

Might it be that our lives are initiated by the sheerest of accidents—the accident of birth, for even if parents "plan" a pregnancy and having a baby, it is only "a" baby that can be planned, never the unique individual that eventually emerges. Every baby is a stranger at the beginning. Thereafter, of course, when we reach a certain age and maturity we begin to choose, whatever it may be, trivial or serious, and we know that our choices make us responsible for them and their detectable consequences. If I choose to do something, it is always choosing that *rather than* something else, and thus I can be held accountable for my decision. Clearly, Jim and Sue chose in some sense to make love one night, and they did that without using the usual sorts of protection, doubtless without giving much thought to outcomes, results, or consequences. But this does not in the least mean that they "caused" the twins to have those severe problems, including premature birth. Just how far, however, do choice and responsibility go? You shouldn't smoke or drink alcohol while pregnant. You should ensure prenatal care. But is Sue or Jim responsible for the components and activities of her or his genetic makeup? If one or the other knew in advance that he or she carried some gene that might eventuate in a genetic disease of some sort (whether cystic fibrosis or something carrying even greater chances of occurring), how precisely does this change the character and range of responsibilities?

Consider this, too: in every significant sense, more deeply than getting pregnant, being born at all with whatever initial biological wherewithal it may be is as unchosen as being born "normal," or with the anomalies Seth and Beth suffered from, or for that matter even as mentally retarded or with a genetic syndrome such as achondroplastic dwarfism. On the other side of the matter, though, is something else: what might be said from the perspective of those twins (or the dwarf, the retarded person, or others)? Would they be correct to hold parents responsible for deciding to go ahead with a pregnancy, even though, say, diagnostic tests performed gave them a pretty good idea of what anomalies their babies would likely present? Of course, most often, children are born relatively free from disabling anomalies, and the question of holding someone or something accountable for one's own birth just doesn't come up. Let there be a baby, or twins, with serious problems, though, and the question seems inevitable, as it surely did to Jim and Sue: there are Seth and Beth, and they did absolutely nothing to deserve their problems, yet the problems are there in living Technicolor. Mustn't someone or something be responsible when something terrible like this occurs? Are their parents then responsible for what happened: their anomalies and premature deaths? We have a sense of the delight in one sense of the "accident of birth," only then to stand back in horror at the other side, when things go wrong and bad things happen to innocent babies. The accident of birth is one thing when all's well; when things go wrong, it's another thing entirely.

Which seems, all things considered, at best scandalous—scandalous just because it seems profoundly unfair, unjust, just not right that such terrible things yet happen, and we can find no one and nothing to blame.[4] In Simon Mawer's complexly ironic novel, *Mendel's Dwarf*, the main character, Ben Lambert (a dwarf who is both the great-great-great nephew of the famous geneticist, Gregor Mendel, and a famous genetic scientist in his own right), succeeds in sequencing the genes which, incorporating a trivial error in a single base pair in "this enigmatic, molecular world," in all likelihood eventually resulted in his being a dwarf. It is, he discovers, a "simple transition at nucleotide 1138 of the *FGFR3* gene."[5] Triggered by one among millions of sperm that once erupted from his father's orgasm that sent them wriggling into the dark recesses of his mother's womb—some of them by chance falling behind and losing, others by chance moving on until finally, one and, in his case, only one was by chance permitted entrance by her ovum (there are chemical attractions and repulsions)—a new life was begun: Ben. And this tiniest of tiny human creatures, this new life began then to divide and divide and divide, the eventual mass of cells becoming, if nothing goes awry, an embryo harboring somehow that genetic error, that transition at just that specific nucleotide 1138 of the *FGFR3* gene, that one mistake in the 3.3×10^9 base pairs in Ben's genome—and it all then mutated into *him*.

Something by chance did go awry, and it resulted in a single substitution of guanine for adenine, in the transmembrane domain of the protein. Of all the millions of pairings along those sinewy, snaky threads of deoxyribonucleic acid (DNA) busily replicating and transporting (RNA) the building blocks of life, proteins, a single letter error occurred, by chance mutation—and then there's Ben, that, as he says many times, hideous, misshapen "monster" who, despite everything, loves Jean the librarian and "normal." Jean, likewise an accident but without such "misspellings" in her genome. Jean, who tries mightily to love Ben, too, but in the end tells him, "It just isn't right, Ben, it isn't right"—now what? If all this occurs by sheer chance, if birth really is the outcome of a series of accidents, do "right" or "not right" make any good sense?

Herbert Spiegelberg wrote about these disturbing questions, and his insight helps to make several things a bit clearer. Having no choice in his own birth, not even *that* he will be born, this unique individual his parents named Ben nevertheless gradually emerges from that globally undifferentiated affair, the embryo and later fetus, developing into a baby, and, after several years of parental nurturing, if he's terribly lucky, he reaches a certain age and from then on bears the brunt of being himself, of becoming whatever it is that he eventually becomes. His birth and thus he himself emerge as an accident and result from many still earlier accidental happenings, including that one-in-a-million chance that just that one single sperm came "to fertilize" that one unique ovum, with one or the other of them unknowingly either carrying that "genetic error" or the potential for that embryonic genome to mutate into that dwarf.

We might well ponder, within that accidental substitution of guanine for adenine, was that one so-called error what made Ben *Ben?* And, if there had been no such mutation, would there have ever been Ben, that scientific genius who cracks the genetic code for achondroplastic dwarfism? "Ben," no less than Seth and Beth (indeed, Jim and Sue, and you and me as well), after all, could just as readily and by the same array and course of other chances, *not* have been born, hence not be at all, or, if born, then born without that chance mutation and for any number of chances that are just as incalculable and accidental as that all the normal processes and timings managed to eventuate in a normal birth.

And is this not exactly what "the accident of birth" means—that, no matter what we'd like to believe, there can simply be no blame, nor in a sense even responsibility? Spiegelberg acutely observed that the "accident of birth" is also the purest kind of "moral chance" as well, and whatever I or Ben or Seth or Beth ends up being at our respective births is utterly undeserved. "I" am, just as Ben and each of the twins is, and I am no more entitled by birth to the circumstances of my birth than was Ben or those twins. I am not entitled to me. I am *given* to me, a gift for me to make of whatever I then go on to make of it, through all sorts of still other chances and accidents (whom I happen to have as "teacher," "preacher," "friend," or "enemy").

One of the choices Ben later faces arises when Jean asks him to use his own sperm for her attempt at in vitro fertilization. He knows how to do it and agrees. Later, checking the resulting embryos, Ben performs the needed diagnostic steps and finds that of them, numbers 3, 5, 6, and 7 are unaffected, no misspelling of adenine by guanine. But numbers 1, 2, 4, and 8 show the mutation. Now what? By chance, four normals and four mutations, four dwarfs-to-be if allowed to be at all. His choice. The consequences and ramifications of his choice, his responsibility as well. Tell Jean? Not tell Jean? Implant which embryo?

Isn't there something outrageous here—a genuine instance of "playing God?" Is this what it's like to *be* God, too? Even if we admit that Ben chose one and not another embryo, which he, of course, does (but I won't spoil the entire story), that of itself does not get rid of the bald, brutal fact of the accident of birth, of initial biological conception and birth with its own particular, utterly unchoosable where-withal—nor, of course, his responsibility for his choices. Even during pregnancy, numerous mutations—some potentially devastating, most not—are occurring all the time, accidents one and all, or at least most of them beyond the catch of cause and effect. That the future person cannot be chosen, furthermore, seems to me at heart to be utterly mysterious. But can we in any sense say that God caused Ben to be a dwarf? That God caused Seth's and Beth's massive problems? Even though, as embryos, fetuses, babies, they cannot be said to have deserved any of that? Yet wouldn't the very notion that God cannot be said to have caused those problems be little short of blasphemy?

The scandal? Is it that our lives are so contingent, so chock full of chance? Or, perhaps, is it that neither you nor I, nor anyone of us, can stand being an accident, and we then try so hard, when we think about it at all, to conceal it, oftentimes through wily postulations of transcendence—whether God or gods, demons or forces?

Here, square on, is a fundamental mystery: each of us is without exception in our origins and for much of our subsequent lives *accidental*. What we are, we are "by chance." We choose neither our parents nor our families nor our socioeconomic circumstances, not even our own biological wherewithal. We seem rather simply to find ourselves as this or that at a certain age on this earth, and the sheer fact of being here at all—how and in the way we each happen to be—occurs with a plain throw of the dice, the sheerest of chances. Is this what God really is?

When Ben finds the eight embryos, four like him and four not, note well that he *can* actually choose which embryo to implant and, if all goes well, allow to grow and become a baby. At a key point, Ben is sitting in his laboratory, the eight embryos in front of him in their respective tubes. He is about to decide whether a "protodwarf" or a "normal" embryo will be implanted in Jean's uterus. Is this "playing God?" I'm inclined to think that it is not, that God, if such there truly be, must act differently. Indeed, if there is a power at work at the source of human life, is it not chance? Ben could choose which embryo to implant, or even whether to implant any. Chance, however, is most obviously at play in the selection of one or another combination of genes and which, if any, mutations occur in the course of development. Ben, to the contrary—and the rest of us— "has the possibility of beating God's proxy and overturning the tables of chance." He, and we, can choose, and "wasn't choice what betrayed Adam and Eve?"[6]

I remember going home the night after the final discussion with Jim and Sue. They had asked that I be there when Seth's ventilator was turned off and he was extubated. I agreed, stayed while the act was done, and soon left. How could I possibly stay any longer? Jim and Sue retired to one of the small rooms where others have gone before to be together, grieving together, as one. Several days later, they asked if I could also be present when treatments were withdrawn from Beth, but, though I did see them briefly with Beth, I wasn't able to attend. Or maybe I just couldn't attend. Even so, I remember that uncanny sense after the withdrawal from Seth when I felt the merest whisper of icy feeling tremble through me, taking me back to that time, only a year and a half before, when I watched my own mother dying.

And Seth? Beth? Was that what Jim and Sue went through, witnessing the same dying of each of their twins? Did they feel that trembling, as I had felt, again, caught unaware soon after I had left the unit, and there it was all over again? Did they feel it, too? Holding their babies as they died, each in its turn and for itself. How best to tell this story, this going on and then ceasing into some elsewhere, with neither saccharine sentiment nor self-important exaggeration?

Strange, that sense: my mother's death, those twins, one at the end of a long life, the others not yet having more than barely begun, the one evoking the other, only then to seem inappropriate, yet dreadful? I recall that shudder even as I shouldered away all those questions and feelings and drove into my driveway, geared up to be with my family.

I hope you understand. Perhaps some of you have come to the same realization about those times when you simply have to forget yourself, your feelings, concerns, and dark fears, so that you can focus just on the people—parents like Jim and Sue and, of course, their families and loved ones—who need help getting through tough situations. And, too, that when you or I chance to help someone like Jim and Sue, we also need help.

It has taken me a long time to understand, and then only reluctantly, something about undergoing the urge to help while, at the same time, coming to realize that I also needed someone else's help. Not that the help we need is all that big a deal. Often, it isn't. Just a chance to tell our story, some "monumentally elusive tale we are always trying to get right,"[7] far more significantly, someone to listen as the simple act of telling does its powerful, magically cleansing work.

It may be—it occurred to me as I was trying to write this story— that helping each other, in times like that faced by Jim and Sue, comes only by someone's listening to us, by letting us be and say what we have to be and say, and in whatever way we have to tell it. Maybe there's some sorcery in the telling; all the more, then, in the act of listening, of *letting people be*, in James Agee's memorable words, as be, however and whenever and whoever they might and need to be at that time, in that place, and in those words that told just that story they had to tell. If we can stand in that "cruel radiance of what is," then that may be all the help any of us can expect, and give.

I think I begin to understand more of that now, telling what I and Jim and Sue had to tell, that it may be the only way to hold sway against what is otherwise a desperate and inchoate loneliness, if we can be with one another while witnessing on behalf of those who are dying. Jim and Sue, too, I believe, eventually came into a kind of understanding when they entered into the realization that they had to say what they felt and thought—the necessary beginning of allowing themselves to grieve, of caring for what they had so hoped to become and were, now, left only to themselves.

If grief, in the telling of it and listening to it, is relearning how to be in the world, it is also the beginning of rebuilding the world that's been shattered by loss. If so, it is clear that the language of feeling, of emotion, must come to be in and from the stories we tell, the anecdotes that tell who and what we are. And, with that, I am once again brought back to that stunning idea: we tell stories because that's what we have to do. It's what we're all about. We care for one another with the stories we place in each other's memory; they are our food for thought, and life.

2

When You're Dead Anyway, What's to Live For?[1]

"I know damn well what I want and don't want, and what I don't want is to be hooked up to that damn machine! Not me, no sir! I've done it, I've had it, and I've had it especially with machines and hospitals and doctors, and I've had it with folks like you."

Neither deft nor subtle, he was, and I'm sure remains, unvarnished. What struck me about Tom was not so much his strident refusal of dialysis as the brutal congenital accident that destined this artless man—gentle even though a bit jarring—to face, unasked, a life riddled with disability and its ineluctable sense of impotence, yet marked too by a curious and unaccountable nostalgia, what seemed when I met him a desperate yearning to be *normal*, "like other people."

Now twenty-eight years old, he had been born with spina bifida: a soft bubble of skin covered a lesion on his spinal column known as myelomeningecele. He was paraplegic, and the ventricles in his brain were enlarged as they regularly filled with cerebral-spinal fluid—hydrocephalus. Like other children with this condition who survive and grow, he needed repeated surgeries over the years to replace the shunt that drained the excess fluid in his brain. He had been incontinent since birth, permanently reliant on a bag outside his body to collect his own wastes.

A nephrologist I know, Jim Stanton, had been on call when Tom came into the emergency room early that morning—luck of the draw, he said later—and had thus inherited Tom as his patient. Jim had noted that Tom had been transferred from another hospital primarily because his refusal to be dialyzed was right there in large letters in the accompanying chart. There were, however, a bagful of "other problems," as they were described in the chart. Indeed.

That summer Tom had began to experience severe diarrhea, dehydration, numerous infections, and a malfunctioning bladder, accounting for the many trips to the hospital over the past several years. The past three months alone he had been admitted four times. As if all that were not enough, his kidneys had recently begun to fail, diarrhea and infections continued and were growing more serious, and he had become anemic. Hospitalized once again, brought in by his mother—his father had disappeared early in life—he staunchly refused to have dialysis even though it clearly held out the promise of at least some benefit, even a return to home and possibly to the job he had worked at for some years. Thinking that Tom might be disturbed and anxious, and with the hope that he might then feel less distressed, be clearer, even change his mind, Jim had prescribed an antidepressant.

"That pill ain't gonna change a thing, doc," Tom told Jim. "I know it, and you know it. Over at McFee Hospital, you know, they said I was nuts, 'specially when I told 'em to just take that damn machine and shove it! You know, kinda like that song, shovin' that job, don't need it, don't want it, take it away; I'll have a beer instead. Oh, lordy, how I do want a beer, or one of them cool milk shakes—ever had one of them, doc? Hell, wasn't all that good to begin with, you know, never could do what I wanted anyhow, and now the damn thing's givin' up all told. Bam! Everything's going to pot, you know, my pisser, no grunt, can't get around 'cause I'm too whipped out. And I stink, oh lordy, do I ever stink! Ain't no pill's gonna change that, even if it will, as you say, make me feel better. 'Feel better!' Hell, that's a laugh. How'm I gonna feel better, stuck with *this?*" His gesture toward his useless legs was plain enough.

Jim Stanton, one of the most gentle, caring, sensitive and able physicians I've known, was deeply upset. He knew that Tom would feel better after dialysis, that he would need it for the rest of his life, but it wasn't imperative at that moment. He felt that Tom was neither "nuts" nor unable to make his own decisions.

I knew, too, that Jim believed—deep in his gut, he said often enough over the coffee we'd gotten in the habit of having several mornings each week—that every competent patient had the right to refuse treatment that wasn't beneficial and that no doctor has any business even thinking about overriding that right. The thing was, though, as he later told me about Tom, dialysis would be therapeutic for him. It *would* help.

What troubled Jim was whether this "right to refuse" included treatments that promised benefit, or was it only about procedures that would not help, neither reverse the lethal process nor stop it—so far as he could tell, "that's what that right is all about, isn't it?" The antidepressant, he said, was intended merely to help calm him down some and help him get some much-needed sleep, for he had no doubts that Tom was not psychiatrically depressed. But, without dialysis soon, within a couple of days at most, he'd begin to lose alertness, and then things would get really sticky. Better to help Tom get a grip now than face forced dialysis later.

Tom finally agreed to a mild sedative, to help calm him down. "This is more for you, doc, than for me, you know what I mean?" Tom punched out the words like he was hammering nails, as he swallowed the pill that first afternoon. Things then moved along, without dialysis and without further upset for a couple of days.

Then Jim got a call that took him out of town for the weekend, and he turned Tom's care over to one of his partners, Fred Inovula. In the rush of things, though, Jim had not told Dr. Inovula about Tom's refusal to be dialyzed. That suddenly dawned on him while he was on the airplane, but he also thought that his carefully crafted chart notes spelled it all out, so there shouldn't be a problem. In any case, he told me later, he had confidence in Fred's judgment and felt that he'd do the right thing.

Fred didn't have the chance to do the right thing, however, for he hadn't yet gone through the chart when he received a frantic call from the resident that Tom was close to decompensating, needed dialysis immediately, and would he please come in immediately to take care of things. When Fred arrived, Tom looked awful: the inevitable buildup of toxins in his bloodstream had seen to that and, Fred thought, clearly accounted for Tom's raving about not wanting any "damn machine." To be safe, Fred called a psychiatrist, who concluded that Tom was not lucid enough to know what he was saying.

"Forget all that," the psychiatrist insisted. "You've got to get him on dialysis or you'll lose him. In a couple of days he'll circle the drain for sure."

The nurses raced Tom to the dialysis unit and snaked a catheter into the shunt in his arm. He remained hooked up to the machine for many hours while it cleaned out his toxins. Afterward, reports of his "acting out" and "making quite a fuss" trailing behind him, he was wheeled back to his room where his mother sat anxiously waiting, at once happy and fearful, for she wanted him to make his own decisions but knew what would happen if he stuck to this one. She had sat with him through all the discussions and had said several times that she wanted his wishes respected even while she shuddered at what would then happen.

Tom's mother was not there when Fred looked in on him the next day, Sunday. He was, however, met with Tom's withering glare. And silence. When Fred tried to check his pulse, Tom ripped his arm away, cursed, and turned to the wall. Fred shrugged it off and went out to the nurse's station. The nurse's overnight notes looked fine, so he again sighed to himself about the kind of patients his partner attracted, "just like fly paper," catching the nurse's eye and winking. He opened the chart to write his note, saw Jim's last one before going out of town, peered, and shuddered. "Pt refuses dialysis," Jim had written, "appears to understand consequences. No dialysis."

When Jim returned and saw Tom later that afternoon, livid and scowling, he knew he'd not connected with Fred. There Tom was, alert once again—the treatment had helped. Aggravated didn't begin to describe his mood. Livid, rather, incensed at everything and everybody.

Tom adamantly restated his refusal of dialysis. Jim and Tom's mother both later told me that they were in the same bind as before. Both wanted to respect what they regarded as Tom's competently expressed refusal, but both also knew that dialysis was actually beneficial. They had living proof of it before their very eyes! But they also felt the crunch of that knowledge: Tom would die without dialysis.

What to do? Jim decided to contact me. Now what?

I agreed to stop by. Things were not urgent at that point and I had a report due, so I asked whether he would mind my doing so in a couple of hours. He said that would be fine.

Something about what Jim told me, though, gnawed at me. Mulling it over, I found myself subtly shifted into a much earlier time in another state when I had come to know another desperate but not terminally ill young man who had also resolutely refused treatment—and caused such consternation he became something of a cause célèbre: Donald (later, self-renamed Dax) Cowart, about whom much has been written.[2]

I began to reminisce, again, about the many times I met with Dax, puzzled over his staunch refusal to be treated for the severe, widespread burns caused by the accidental explosion of his car in 1973— the result of a faulty propane gas line at the bottom of the slope where he and his father had stopped to check out a possible real estate transaction that fateful day in 1973 close to the East Texas town where he lived after returning from a tour on active duty in the Air Force. Pilot, former footballer, still active in rodeos, Dax, then twenty-six, had to face a future blind, crippled, fingers gone, and able to walk only short distances at a time. He said "no way," and gave the hospital folks hell for fourteen months before being discharged. Several suicide attempts later, with some control finally over his inability to sleep, he made it through law school so that he could, in some still only dimly imagined future, defend his, and any other patient's right to self-determination. A passionate man. Driven and determined. And amazingly articulate in his own cause. Maybe he should have been more than a merely temporary, minor cause célèbre. Still, his case did in fact play a serious role in subsequent thinking about major moral and legal principles needed to govern a health care system rapidly running ahead of itself and society.

I thought a lot about Dax, at the time and again that day when I heard about Tom. I didn't really want another one of those, even though I had not had to contend with Dax while in the hospital. Is *that* what I would now face here, in this hospital?

Before going to his room, I wanted to look in his chart, as if there might be some clues—if nothing else, notes from the prior hospital—about his "refusal." Mr. Thomas Yarbrough Brown's life had been unfolding—unraveling, more likely—from an infancy I had already encountered many times before in newborn intensive care units (NICUs) and, more recently, in an experimental protocol being conducted in a maternal-fetal unit, seeking to determine whether this type of lesion could be closed in utero and whether that would be beneficial. Both were fascinating and not a little disturbing.

In any case, here I was, now facing Tom. Born with spina bifida, his spinal column was exposed and, in his case, protruded from a large lesion covered by a slight puff of skin (myelomeningocele) at about the third lumbar vertebra. He had undergone surgery soon after birth to close the lesion, though he was pretty much paralyzed from that point down: incontinence, paraplegia, and hydrocephalus were his daily life, and, periodically, he had gone through numerous replacement operations for the shunt in his brain ventricles (infections, becoming displaced, or outgrown). Mr. Thomas Y. Brown had come to know hospitals exceedingly well.

Severe diarrhea. Dehydration. Malfunctioning bladder. In addition, in the last month or so his kidneys were failing. His renal disease was thought to be end stage and irreversible, although not untreatable; hemodialysis had worked for him over some years, and a kidney transplant could be effective. The diarrhea and infections were difficult to treat, and, as they continued, he had become anemic.

On the admissions form in the chart was the information Jim had mentioned to me—the refusal of dialysis, that he might be "distressed, if not depressed" (prompting Jim to prescribe the mild antidepressant, hoping that, if he were less distressed, he might change his mind), and his many illnesses prior to winding up in our emergency room. Despite what I had inferred from Jim's description, Tom still might be unclear about that demand to be left alone—whether it was the gradual buildup of toxins in his blood, some reaction to one of his many medications, the suffering he experienced in a lifetime of problems, or a genuine, clear-cut, competent, and irrevocable choice.

The chart also indicated that his mother, divorced from his father for many years, had accompanied him to the hospital. There were apparently no brothers or sisters. According to a nurse's note the day of his admission, Mrs. Brown obviously expected that he would be put on dialysis. Perhaps, she mentioned to the nurse, he might even "get one of those kidneys from someone, you know?" It was something their family doctor had brought up one time, she pointed out. Her son's refusal to be dialyzed was clearly deeply disturbing to her.

When I read his chart, my first thoughts were of all the babies I had seen in the NICU. It was as if one of them had suddenly grown up and was now demanding to know why he had been forced to stay alive. I recalled one mother insistently demanding of the neonatologist treating her damaged premature baby: "It's just not right to force my baby to be a hero, to make him live the only life he'll be able to live, all crippled and spending half his life in hospitals. That's not fair!" It probably wasn't "fair," not in the least. But, despite that, what could be done?

Until the time of this consult, I had enjoyed the luxury of merely listening to those sad entreaties, musing more idly than actively about what the future held for this or any of the other many babies with spina bifida. Now, it seemed, here that future was, in Technicolor, in the very specific person of Mr. Thomas Yarbrough Brown.

It was as if my earlier musings had abruptly come alive: what would I do were I actually to meet him? Embarrassed by what bubbled up unwanted in my fancy, I found myself face to face with something none of us would like to admit, surely not openly: that certain sort of embarrassment and dismay, even awkward aversion, toward disabled persons. This, despite the fact that a seriously handicapped person has been my best friend for many years.

Still, guardedly noticing these feelings, most unwanted and not a little discomfiting by themselves, and realizing this about myself, at least gave me the opportunity to be more alert for some of those subtle ways these most often skillfully buried attitudes play out in surprising ways—startling ourselves most, if we dare admit it. I also suspected that, when I eventually would meet him, Mr. Brown would doubtless not be much like what I expected.

Which was true in spades. Soon after looking over his medical chart, I went into his room. He seemed to be asleep. His mother was sitting next to his bed and looked up as she heard me enter. I said hello and introduced myself. Before I could say anything else her son opened his eyes, looked at me and said, "Hey, man, I'm Tom"— and the image of all those spina bifida babies whose fates I had so often wondered about, feared too, dissolved. Tom looked and sounded so *normal*.

"Mr. Brown? I'm Dr. Zaner . . ."

"*Another* one? How many of you are they going to send in here anyway? I've said all I'm going to say, and that's that . . ."

"Now, Tom, Tommy, please don't be rude, not again, not now," his Mom exclaimed.

"Mom, I've told you, I'm fed up, and here they are sending another damned doctor in to try and talk me out of it . . ."

"Mr. Brown, please let me finish: I'm not 'another one of *them*,' as you obviously think; I'm not a physician, and I'm not about to try and talk you into or out of anything . . ."

"Then what the hell are you?"

"Tommie," his mother cut in quickly, "watch your tongue!"

"OK, Ma, OK. So what and who are you then, Mr. Dr. whatever?"

I tried a small smile with a few words to match: "I'm not so sure, now that you ask. I'm not sure you've ever heard of people like me before: I'm in ethics, and I'm supposed to try and help you, your mother, and the doctors see if there is some way this impasse, this blockade about dialysis, can be . . ."

Encouraged by the way he looked at me, I sat down in a chair, prepared now to do what I knew I had to do: talk about his refusal of dialysis, and therefore about death. This, it seemed to me, was the matter that both he and his mother needed to think about together and discuss at length. I had earlier wondered whether they had ever done much thinking and talking about what would inevitably happen should he not be treated. Now, I still wasn't sure just how best to bring up that matter. Did he know that refusing treatment would mean *his* death? Did his mother understand that? Is there some sort of guilt, maybe resentment, all caught up in the midst of this confrontation with his doctors and his mother?

After that brief exchange and a quick glance at his mother, to see if she was listening, I turned back to Tom with the idea of just going at the issues directly, opening up the question of death, maybe backing off a bit should he react strongly, but going directly to the point rather than avoiding and evading like, I felt, he must have come across many times in his life.

But as I began his eyes rolled up, only the whites showing, his face contorted, his arms stiffened, then heaved up, one jerked knocking the coverlet off the bed, his body going into spasms. He twitched and jerked. His mother quickly picked up the coverlet, turned to him, touched his brow, his arm, murmured words I couldn't hear. His withered legs were partially exposed when the coverlet fell off, and her face was marked with apprehension and concern.

She looked up at me, pleading, and I quickly backed out: "I'll get the nurse." I stared at his writhing body and wondered whether or how I could have brought that on, realizing how stupid is the very thought, when a nurse came by. "He's having another seizure," she said, which was the first I'd heard of this. Jim sure didn't let me in on very much.

He spasmed and convulsed, and I tried to unsay what I had just said, thinking without thinking: What in the world does ethics have to do with this? I tried to unwalk my way back out again but was trapped by his mother's pleading glance; it pinned me down. When she pulled back to stare at her son writhing on the bed, relief flooded over me. Yet, I, too, was drawn back to look, gape really, at him, wanting to help, realizing there's nothing I could or should have done, just stay out of the way of the nurse, savior to us all. She glided in and around me as I dodged and finally crept out.

Keeping some presence of mind, I apologized to his mother and promised to come back the next day. I doubt she heard me, so focused was she on her son's lurching torso as it lifted up the sheets, head snapping side to side, and I inadvertently caught a glimpse of a massive chest and solid shoulders, but legs shriveled from the hips down. I left.

This was the first time I had ever witnessed a grand mal seizure in person, and I found myself badly shaken. I found myself wondering, oddly, whether I had caused his seizure. As I later learned, most of those taking care of Tom had been so centered on his refusal of dialysis that nobody, attending included, had remembered to mention the seizures and the fact that, after years of being effectively controlled, they had recently returned. As if everything else that he had endured over the past months were not enough, now he had to contend with that.

Thinking about that, his refusal readily, though perhaps also mistakenly, took on greater weight. Realizing that such "natural" tendencies can be just as "naturally" misleading, even quite "unnatural,"

I worked to mute the inclination, as I wandered off down the hallway preoccupied with such notions and feelings both fleeting and palpable. So much so, I was later told, rather bluntly, I failed even to notice the chaplain or hear her greeting. Just walked right by.

The next morning I came back to see Mr. Brown and his mother. They were both much calmer.

"As I started to say yesterday, Mr. Brown . . ."

"Why don't you just call me 'Tom'? Everyone else does, and it is my name, you know? He explained how uncomfortable he was with "Mr." this or "Mrs." that.

"Fine with me, but only if you use my name, too: I'm 'Dick.' I'm concerned with ethics in the hospital," but I was quickly interrupted again by what I took to be a rebuff.

"Ethics? Well, I've heard of folks like you, but never thought I'd meet one." Despite everything, he actually smiled.

"A rare opportunity, then, right? Play it to the hilt, Tom, 'cause you may never get another chance!"

"Oh, don't worry, Dr. Dick, I will, 'specially if you can keep these docs' hands off a me!"

What do you say to that? Right from the mouth itself! The better part of wisdom counseled to ignore that, now, and get on with what I had come to find out.

"Actually, Tom, I would have thought you'd not be in the least surprised at my being here, what with you refusing to be dialyzed. You must know that caused your doctors no end of dismay, shock even."

"You like to use the big words, don't you? Well, never mind, maybe I'm not well-educated, but I can follow you, but just don't start talking down to me."

"Tom," I began again refusing to take the bait, "I know that you don't want to be dialyzed."

"Damn straight," he said. You could almost see him stomp on the point. "And they'd better not do it again, like happened a couple of days ago, you know about that?"

"I heard about it, Dr. Stanton told me, in fact. But maybe we should talk about all that—not about the dialysis you got on Saturday, but about what you want, why you've said you don't want to be treated now. You know, you've really got folks around here up in the air, not knowing just what to make of you, of your refusing to be treated. Have you thought about that?"

"You ever been hooked up to one of them?"

"No, Tom, I haven't, but . . ."

"Well, you just try it sometime, see what you think."

"I'm not the one needing dialysis, Tom. You are, and I just want to listen to what you understand about that, and what will happen if you are not treated. Has Dr. Stanton discussed this with you and your mother?"

"Well, sure, he's talked some, but, hell, he hasn't had to have it done, either, so what's he know what it's like?"

"He's very experienced in his field and has been with a lot of patients, Tom. While he's never been dialyzed, he knows a lot about it and about how patients feel about it. Anyway, you have discussed it with him?"

"Well, yeah, some, 'bout ever time he comes in here. Ma though, she don't like to hear suchlike, do you Ma? So, he don't like to talk much while Ma's here."

I looked over at his mother, but her eyes were downcast, her eyes closed, or so it seemed. Was she asleep? Was she taking any of this in? I'd have to find out, but then, Tom kept on; he did like to talk, I had to admit, even to admire, given the circumstances.

"But, damn, what am I supposed to do? All I been doing the past several years is going to some damned hospital or other, getting this and that, and after all that I still feel awful. I'm just so God-awful tired of it all, don't you know? Wouldn't you be?"

He was obviously someone of not inconsiderable intelligence, a person fond of banter and even irony, but nonetheless I refused again to take this bait, turning instead directly to his mother. Although I had tried to include her in the conversation, she hadn't said anything and was still looking down. "Were you in on the talks with Dr. Stanton, Mrs. Brown?"

She was very alert, it turned out.

"Well, just once, right after Tom was brought here from that other hospital. But it was all confusing, and things were in such a rush. He talked, just a little, 'cause he was busy and all. Other times, I wasn't here."

Did either of them understand the full implications of his refusal of dialysis? In a way, as we continued to talk Tom seemed to, but it became pretty clear to me that he hadn't really thought about it very well. While we talked, he seemed very different from what you'd expect when meeting someone firmly refusing potentially life-saving treatment. Not that he was calmly acceptive of the decline and death that would inevitably follow if he weren't dialyzed, just that he seemed not to have confronted it at all squarely. The thought that he would die without dialysis had, so to speak, sort of sidled past his awareness now and then, but he had not faced matters directly. He had not in fact discussed the matter with his mother, nor had she made her own feelings explicit with him, had not really even thought about it much herself.

I couldn't say, not yet, that he was in any sense "ready" to accept his own death (Is anyone ever ready?) for when I turned to his mother—she had just been sitting there, saying nothing—he grew visibly anxious. Not only had he not discussed the matter with his mother, nor had she raised the issue with him, he had not really even thought about it much for himself. When I asked about advance directives, he seem only puzzled at first, before he saw the point and acknowledged that he had not signed any advance directive; the idea hadn't even occurred to him. It was obvious that neither knew much about, much less had considered, advance directives or the clear consequence of his refusal.

As best as I could tell in that moment, the thought that he would die without dialysis had just sort of floated past his awareness now and then, but he had not confronted matters squarely. Nor had she made her own feelings explicit with him.

"Oh, I tried several times to talk about what he's doing to himself, to me, you know, about maybe he should think about all that some . . ."

"Ma, I done told you, I don't want to hear about all that."

"See, Dr. Zaner, that's the sort of . . ."

"Ma, like I said, why don't you just hush now! I told you how many times, I don't like that kind of talk."

I had wandered onto some very sensitive ground, so I thought it might be better to shift directions. I didn't want to lose him, or his mother. Besides, knowing so very little about him personally, I thought it would help if I tried to repair my ignorance, to learn more about him and his life. I asked him what he did, did he have a job?

"Oh yeah, man! I've got a *good* job. 'Least I *had* a damned good job . . ." His voice trailed off. He looked up at me, looking nothing so much like a wounded deer waiting denouement. Then, he looked back down, it seemed to me, at the bulge his useless legs made in the bed sheet. Then he began again.

"I work—better to say, I worked—in the main office of the state office where disabled folks are evaluated and money's handed out when they need it, for food and rent and suchlike. Really like it, too. I got to the point where I was promoted and able to do a bunch on my own, you know, like they say, real independence, not only at work but outside, too. Fact, I was right on the edge of trying to get me an apartment for myself, close to the building where I work, still'd see Ma, 'course, but . . ." His voice trailed off again.

Clearly, he enjoyed his work—or the fact that he had a job, that he could work at all—enormously. And he took considerable pride in it all, apparently for the way the disabled could get help, him having a part in that. Now, it was just as obvious that he was deeply suffering over having apparently lost it.

To keep him talking to me, I decided to get into another side of his life, so I asked about his childhood, school, and such. He brightened some, then his voice picked up. He had lived with his mother since birth, and she had taken care of him the entire time, all through elementary and high school. Obviously, he loved her and, as I glanced over at her, she, too, had perked up as he chatted on about his childhood, her taking care of him, "wheelin' me all 'round and about," as he said. A note of pride crept in. She, too, brightened, her eyes riveted on him. Obviously, she felt very, very close to him, cared deeply for him. Even, he pointed out with some pride, during the two years he went to night school, while he worked during the day. She nodded, remembering, "Them were good days, Tommie, good days, weren't they?"

"Oh, yeah, like I said, I'm not too educated, but Ma did see to it that I got around a good bit. I even did that accounting course, 'cause of my job, remember Ma?"

She nodded, began to rise, then sat back, silent again. Her brow dark, eyes clouded.

The reminder of those times brought him out of his funk, a bit anyway, even if it brought her down, remembering then, seeing now.

"Before I got so sick some time back," he quietly mused, "I had begun to think that I might, finally, after all these years get me an apartment and begin to live on my own; I know I can do it. Hell, I cook some right now at home, don't I Ma?"

"Oh, yes, Dr. Zaner . . ."

"Please, Mrs. Brown, use my name, 'Dick,' OK?"

"I appreciate it, sir, but I'm just not real comfortable doing that; I guess I'm just of the old school when it comes to that."

"Well, whichever you prefer. Just keep in mind, I don't mind."

"Anyway," Tom continued, "I almost got me that apartment, had one located, remember, Ma?"

"Mmm, yes, but I don't rightly recall where it was."

"Down on Seventh, and near enough I could wheel on down to work and home. Rain? Ice? Never mind, I'd figure it out."

That, it dawned on me as he talked—his voice, but also his demeanor spoke volumes—was what was really on his mind. Glancing over at his mother, her look confirmed that she, too, saw this.

"It just got so's I couldn't keep up the job, being in and out of the hospital so much, you know? I just couldn't get much work done. There were times when I was out more'n a week."

He wound down, noting that the many illnesses and hospitalizations, he thought, made it necessary for him to quit, though he hadn't discussed this with anyone, at least not with his mother. This, more than anything else, seemed to me the source of what had been labeled his "depression." Like any of us at one time or another, he had then gone on to "figure it all out" for himself. On dialysis two or three times a week, four or five hours each session, he would not be able to hold down any job, much less go back to the one he really liked, and the apartment? Forget it, that was out: no paycheck, no apartment. Ergo, life isn't worth it, might as well be dead anyway, so just give it up!

Being *normal*—working and living independently—had become insurmountable at the very time when it seemed for the first time actually in reach, as he now looked at things from his hospital bed. I listened as he continued talking, softly remembering how things used to be, how they might have been, but no longer, not now, not ever.

"You know, Dr. Z," he went on, musing, and with the change in my name, I noted also a subtle shift in his mood, "I really liked that job, really liked what I was doing, the other people there, and it's worthwhile, lord knows I know that! Helping folks like me, man, that really came to mean something heavy, you know?"

"I'm sure it did, Tom. But did you really have to quit?"

"Well, a few months ago," he said, almost as an afterthought, "I talked with Mrs. Johnson—she's my supervisor—and . . ." His voice faded off. "We talked about all that," he began to pick up again, "and I told her what with all that going in and out of hospitals, and dialysis and suchlike, I didn't rightly know how I could keep it up, you see, how I could keep it up. Didn't seem at all fair, don't you know, to the other folks there, there being a policy that nobody gets treated special 'cause they're crippled or whatever. No special treatment, even the book said that . . ." and again he faded out.

"Tom," his mother broke in, "didn't you tell me the other day that you'd had another talk with Mrs. Johnson, on the phone, wasn't it, while you were at that, at McFee that last time? 'Course, you were terrible sick that time, don't you know. But didn't I tell you that she'd called, and don't you recall you'd talked with her? I know you said how it weren't fair to the others there, nor the disabled and suchlike, but I thought you'd finally gotten around to calling her back and talking some, hadn't you?"

"Oh, lord, yes," Tom, now becoming animated, "Mrs. J, that's what she wants us to call her, she, oh my lord, she told me that I could still have the job, after I got well again. But I just couldn't get well enough to be there all the time they needed me. I just couldn't get back to work, and . . ."

As soon as he said this he perked up. His speech became more spirited, his gestures more lively.

"That's right," his mother quickly affirmed, "Mrs. Johnson . . ."

"Mrs. J, Mom . . ."

". . . Did say you could have your job back when you're able. It was just that you couldn't get able enough."

"But how can I work?" Tom's tremulous words seemed at once hopeful and wary, "when I've got to be on that damned machine so much? Besides going in and out of all these damned hospitals!"

"Tommie, just please shush such awful words now, hear?"

"OK, OK, Ma, still . . ."

At this point his mother and I vied with each other to get the thing said: work was indeed possible. Hadn't he discussed this with his doctor? He wasn't sure. Perhaps he had been so wrapped up in grief and a deep sense of loss that he hadn't heard; perhaps none of his doctors mentioned it, or, if any of them had, Tom hadn't heard, hadn't understood.

In any event, it was by now clear that the way things appeared had changed dramatically for him. As his chart had indicated, he had begun to improve somewhat over the past month or so. His last hospital stay seemed to have helped. His anemia was getting under control, too. I suggested that he really needed to find out, really to understand, much more about his many medical problems. For that, he just had to talk directly and pointedly with Dr. Stanton, especially about dialysis and whether he could arrange to have it done in the evenings and, since he hadn't talked with Mrs. Johnson, he needed to do so right away to see if he would still be able to return to work and when he might do that.

The conversation wound down. It was perfectly obvious that the young man causing so much disturbance among hospital staff was no longer there, but had abruptly left, replaced by what Mrs. Brown described as "the ol' Tommie." He did not want to refuse dialysis. If he could work, which is what he desperately wanted to do, get back to work. For that, it was necessary to set up meetings with his doctor who would be able to help him arrange a convenient place for outpatient treatment and, eventually perhaps, be evaluated for a transplant.

Walking again into Tom's room, I found myself undergoing an experience as fascinating as it is transformative. I've noted many times how everything in such rooms is *oriented* in very specific and powerful ways: glances, talk, gestures, equipment, attention, all are focused around and directed to Tom. This is in striking contrast to the structural imbalance of the relationship he ineluctably has with Dr. Stanton and the other doctors and nurses and others, maybe even me—these relationships are *asymmetrical* with power on our side, not Tom's. His physician, for example, not Tom, has the knowledge and skills to help, has access to resources (diagnostic technologies, prescription drugs, surgeons, hospitals, and all the rest) and is legally authorized and socially legitimated to use his knowledge and skills for Tom—and, of course, all his patients. Not only is Tom compromised by illness, but he is also disadvantaged by the very relationship to the people (doctors, nurses) who profess the ability to help him.

Nevertheless, entering his room, it becomes increasingly evident that there is another kind of imbalance here. Tom is a presence, and he dominates the room. He is the center of attention, the hub of all activity. Thinking about this, it also occurs to me that these notions—being oriented by Tom's presence and his being the center of attention and action—are complex in ways that can be delineated, spelled out.

Simply lying there in that bed, he is compelling and exercises a peculiar attraction for anyone who comes into his room. It's a realization that is set in motion already by going into the hospital itself. It is almost as if he embodies a kind of magnetism or gravity that pulls glances, gestures, actions, and talk toward him. A feeling comes over me that I want to, even must, do or say *something*. At the same time, even as I am drawn to him I also sense that I am, oddly, intrusive—even though I may have been invited or, because of my duties, "belong" there—as if the mere act of my looking at him were somehow a trespass on forbidden or at least vulnerable terrain: *be careful!* seems as if announced by the very air. This feeling remains with me until he indicates that it's OK: he says "hello," and I'm able to go on. Still, it's as if talk takes, or verges on taking, the shape of apology—a preliminary asking to excuse the trespass, a breaking into pain or awareness fogged by drugs. But even with permission, it's hard to know just what to say, and how to say it. Why is this?

Exposed and vulnerable, Tom is a sort of dialectical opposite to the usual sense of gravity or force of attraction: he *attracts* my notice, he attracts *my* notice, he draws my looks, concern, words, and actions toward himself, precisely by and through the *difference* he embodies from a positive force. His vulnerability, while in a sense a kind of "negative" (openness to manipulation, for instance), is yet potent and positive. There is a vibrancy, an aliveness that is sensed in the way people usually appear: the look of his eyes (welcoming, threatening), the lift of her flesh (face, hands, movements), or the spoken word (pauses, emphases). This aliveness is muted in illness, even when, as with Tom, pain or seizure drives sudden spasms, forceful gestures, and bodily displays across his face and torso. Grievously ill, even if treatable, Tom's body has a pallor, a kind of wanness that provokes wonder: is he himself still vibrantly present within that body? Even when he seizes?

Tom's vulnerability is clear and unmistakable: abed, begowned, seizing, monitors and tubes haloed around him. Yet the exposure that leaves any patient open and readily available for medical examination, nursing ministration, and various technical soundings (auscultation) and touchings (palpation) is commanding and compelling. You feel it immediately on entering Tom's room: *Don't touch! Watch what you say! Wash your hands! Don't sneeze!*

This vulnerability itself attracts, directs anyone who approaches a patient to *be careful* in words, touches, glances. In front of the sick person we seem as if dragged out of ourselves—my own concerns seem so petty—and drawn toward and by the other, the one who is sick or injured. What can or could be done to him is silently governed by a potent and rigorous form of *restraint*. Ancient physicians termed this *sophrosyne* and, blended with *dike* (justice or judgment), understood these as the prime virtues of the "art." But anyone who enters Tom's room feels, along with the magnetism, a kind of temptation of one's gaze by Tom, a sort of alluring restraint or constrained fascination along with concern—it's hard to get the right words for this—when encountering him: "Look at him, lying there. Look at those shoulders, see those withered legs!" There is, too, a temptation having an almost physical jolt: how easy it would be to take control of this vulnerable person, how open and exposed he is for . . . sexual advance, torture, deceptive eliciting for a research project, or simply anything the one who has the edge of advantage may want.

Yet, at the same time, I sense an equally demanding responsibility I can't step around, can't avoid at the very least noticing (so that ignoring it is a choosing to ignore it): *never* take advantage of the sick person, *precisely because* he is sick. Vulnerability augurs temptation but at the same time evokes—seems even to awaken—concern, a wanting to care. It entices seduction but also compels respect. It foreshadows swift action, but caution, too. And it invites being oblivious and heedless to this specific individual, Tom, though, at the same time evokes singular sensitivity to hurts and harms he is already undergoing and suffering and those you could cause.

In this specific way, Tom, like most any sick person, awakens an otherwise mostly dormant moral sense. Facing Tom in his room is compelling, though I know, too, that I could also just walk out of there, or could take advantage of his weakened condition, and so on. Instead, I experience just that complex sense evoked by his vulnerability and that paradoxical temptingness and yet respect. My encounter with Tom is precisely one of those remarkable but rare occasions when, entering such rooms, I've found myself subtly taken over by that sense that, now, being here and not elsewhere, I've come into a special kind of responsibility, one that cannot be gainsaid.

These feelings, moreover, invariably have specific *focus:* there is a kind of mindfulness that is *directed to* the sick person ("How do you feel?"); feelings are *oriented toward* the patient's particular circumstances ("What's wrong with you?") and *aimed at* his or her possible futures ("When will you get better?"). This affective ground, if you will, is almost visceral in the way alertness is drawn to and by the sick person—it's an almost tangible tug that I must now *be mindful* of Tom, here and now, within the actual context of his compelling vulnerability (not to mention the vulnerability evidently tied to his mother's being in the room).

These feelings propel me *beyond* myself, take me out of myself, beyond my own concerns of the moment, *toward* Tom. They are an elemental and literal *ec-stasis;* to be myself before Tom is to be beyond myself, always already with him. I find myself busied with *him*, not me. Being myself, as it were, is something I have to accomplish within these very circumstances: it is with Tom that I am brought to myself; "self," more a prize won through complex developmental experiences than some "inside" entity brooding in me. Thus is understandable that otherwise odd sense of gratitude one feels in being able to help someone like Tom, even if it is merely to have placed a full glass of water next to him as he asked.

These feelings are, as it were, "*come upon*"—they happen to or in me, not that I set about to activate, "feel," them—in that I in no way produce them out of whole cloth, nor do I decide to feel this or that way. Rather, I find myself feeling this way. Sensing them, I seem more to find myself in their grip than to plot or plan them out ahead of time. It's not even proper to say, "I feel," as it is rather a matter of "something is felt in and by me." With Tom, I simply found myself sensing feelings and thoughts bubbling up from some sort of subterranean bed, many of them retrospectively embarrassing: "What's it like to be—what *is* it, trapped?—in that body?" "There but for the grace of God go I!" *Really?* Is my life, is Tom's life, *chance?* Are we each who we are only . . . by chance? Luck of the draw? *Bona fortuna?* What, then, is God?

Tom's presence there, in that bed, that room, this hospital—this *ecstatic* moment, pulling me out of myself and into concern for him, his sphere of life—is deeply embedded and inscribed in my life. He remains there, lodged. I had the sense then, and still have it now, that his being sick is what does this, and contributes to what I, this self, am. For that, for what in addition he taught me to see—about him, his mother, other matters—I am grateful.

What gradually came into focus as I talked with him, and later as I reflected on that encounter, also has to do with his being in that body—paraplegic, large if doughy shoulders, that grimacing face, flared nostrils, writhing torso—which in this moment seems a profoundly unjust, even macabre dance, as if he were possessed: that seizure. Yet, I knew and know better.

But what is that body of his? Does he experience it in much the way I experience mine: at times frustrating; happy compliance at others? That organism, it embodies Tom as mine embodies me. But what is this, that "intimate union" that has frustrated so many since Descartes seemed to split it all asunder in trying to lift up our puny lives into universal truths? Yet paradoxically always seeking, as he did, in the name of health, of medicine! So intimate is Tom bound to his embodying body, as I am to mine, that there is the constant temptation to say, he *is* that body; hit *my* body and you hit *me*. Where my body is, I am also. Is this how and where that strong, primal sense of belonging begins? Here, within my own relation to my own body, Tom to his?

Yet, although the relation between Tom and Tom's body is deeply intimate, just like my own, I think, does he also experience his oddly formed body as strange and alien, in the way it seems strange and alien to me? Do I really know all that goes on in it? I don't make my hair grow, my bowels churn up food, my blood flow: are these *mine*, too, as is my arm, my head, my ideas, myself? Is this true as well for Tom? What must it be like to have his body?

Tom's body, like mine and yours, seems at the source (though not the only part of that) of what ethics is all about; it is, was, just what made my encounter with him so puzzling and difficult. On the other hand, the profound moral feelings evoked by certain medical practices (dialysis, transplantation, chemotherapy) and almost any experimentation (for instance, cloning, genetics, fetal surgery) are understandable, as they are precisely ways of intervening or intruding into that most intimate and integral of regions: my own, your own, Tom's own, body. In whatever other sense Tom is alive, he is surely alive in that his body, what he experiences at the base of all he does, feels, thinks—in that his body is alive.

Tom was and continues to be inscribed, to dwell within me (as he does within all those who cared for and took care of him), part of what I have become since meeting and talking with him. The relationship between Tom and me is deeply *reflexive*. Kierkegaard was right: the reflexive is at the heart of being a self. Even in our language, the word "self" is reflexive, an expression divested of the pronominative it modifies (my-self, your-self, our-selves, them-selves, its-self). Seeing Tom is seeing Tom seeing me. Hearing him, I hear myself and know myself hearing him. Touching his hand, I at once touch and am touched—in multiple ways. He and I are reflexively related to each other and to ourselves, as are his mother and I when I turn to her and ask if it's OK for me to come back tomorrow and she says, "Sure, do that." We each talk and listen simultaneously to ourselves and to each other.

Trying to figure out who Tom really is is incredibly slippery and complex; the same is true of me or you. Even more so is figuring out the relationship between two such slippery and complex creatures! Tom casts knowing looks at his mother when she chides him for cursing. She sinks further into sadness (look at her eyes and mouth, witness even her cheeks) when she hears him talk about his death. As Tom relates to his mother, he does so within the awareness that I am there and watching: he sometimes performs for me, as I do for him. He notes her reaction/relation/response to him; and she, reacting to his cursing, knowing I too am there hearing it, chiding him, notes his reaction/relation/response to her.

This is a wonderful game, going on not only between people well known to each other, but among strangers. Note merely how you and some stranger (most often) adroitly maneuver around each other in a crowded terminal, even though we both are preoccupied with other matters. Tom and I are talking to each other; each of us relates to, experiences, and values the other ("I like what you said, Tom, but . . ."); each of us relates to, experiences, and values himself within the relationship to the other (I'm beginning to feel good about myself as I listen to him talk about his job; maybe I helped him get to this point, I think to myself); and each of us relates reflexively to, experiences, and values the relationship itself (we conclude, saying to each other that the discussion was a good one).

Encountering Tom, I had the sense of entering into, coming upon, or "happening" onto something that seemed then and now terribly significant, saturated with values, obligations, responsibilities, character traits, virtues, the works. The ground of ethics seems closely bound up with just that form of reflexive relatedness to and with the other person—perhaps most poignantly presented in view of my entering his personal sphere as a stranger. We didn't know each other, and thus had nothing on which to base expectations or beliefs, beyond the usual, the typical, the common.

Illness itself is a strangeness. Tom knew and knows this well. Even while I am, of course, familiar with what it's like to be sick or injured—from my own experience, from what I learned from others—to come upon Tom in this way, I find myself ineluctably facing multiple unknowns and challenges. Tom is at once a challenge and an appeal. Although he is not terminally ill, he certainly verges on that when he says "no more dialysis," because of which the scene between us is set up in even more dramatic ways.

Who, what, are you now, Tom? What can or should I do to help you and your mother? How should I act toward you? Do you really mean what you say about dialysis? What should I say? Standing bodily, boldly, before you as someone who may well be dying, and I don't know you, what can you do to help me help you? Or, do you want my help at all?

Perhaps all that can and even should be done is simply to be there: seeing each other, touching hands, feeling that rough skin on my palm, talking together, watching each other, talking with "Ma," joshing with the nurse, and we do all of this without ever taking much note of it so much as just sensing that things are better this way. If you are dying, Tom, the notion ran through me, maybe these simple gestures are all I can do, but they, like your gestures toward me, are precisely what they are, no more nor less, which may be their magic: affirmations of each other as worthwhile, worth the time. You make a difference. You matter, Tom.

When I first entered into Tom's life, when I "came upon" him the day after that awful seizure, it gradually dawned on me how vividly present we had already become to one another, despite how short and temporary the relationship. It was as if, knowing that I had witnessed his seizure, he now saw me has having shared some dark but precious secret. We, Tom and I, had already begun to matter to each other.

The last time I visited Tom he was, as he said, "hooked"—he loved to play on that metaphor—to the dialysis machine. He shared with me that his boss had told him he could have his old job back; it was there when he was ready. He was very upbeat and planned on going back to work within a couple of days. He joshed about the machine, joked with his nurse, and offered again to come to one of my classes and talk about himself.

For whatever reason, I didn't ask him why he had earlier refused to be precisely where he was now. Nor can I ask him now; that seems just too intrusive. Maybe later, when he has (or I have) had time to think about and live with things, when time can work its subtle alchemistry on both of our memories and deepest feelings about ourselves. Then, perhaps, I can ask. But, then, don't I already know?

I'm not sure why Tom still remains so firmly in my mind. It's not so much his refusal, though that stands out for me today, as it is the harsh accident of his birth and the turmoil of his life. That utterly fortuitous and sly genetic accident that destined this gentle, guileless man to face, unasked, a life marked by curious nostalgia for what he could only guess at, yearning to be like the rest of us, never quite realizing that he might not want that at all, not at all.

3

Hope against Hope[1]

A seventy-two-year-old woman, Mrs. Oland, had been hospitalized for over four months. She had been married for forty-nine years to a gentle, caring man several years her senior and in good health. They had raised three children, now adults, two of whom lived outside the city in which Mrs. Oland was hospitalized. Their daughter, Janice, was married to a successful local real estate broker and continues to live in the same city not far from her parents. She often served as caretaker for either of them, when needed, and visited them at home several times a week.

Regular visitors to the hospital included Mr. Oland, Janice and her brother, the eldest, Charlie, who did well in a construction business in another city, within easy driving distance. The other daughter, Jenny, remained unmarried, working as a legal secretary in a city far away. She was unable to visit often and had been to see her mother during the lengthy hospital stay only once.

Mrs. Oland had been diagnosed with several serious illnesses, any one of which could be life threatening: prolonged hypotension, recurrent pneumothorax (air in her pleural cavity), respiratory failure, and end-stage renal disease. Her attending physician for the current admission, Dr. Stanley Langston (a nephrologist who has not treated her before), noted in her medical chart that her prognosis was "dismal." This conclusion was consistent with those of the various consultants he had called in to help manage her multiple medical problems, as well as fitting with what he had been told by her primary physician, Dr. Fred Copple, who had known Mrs. Oland for many years.

She was not expected to recover renal function or to be weaned from the ventilator. She managed to eat normally for a few days, but as her alertness faded because of the kidney problems, she was unable to take in sufficient nutrition by mouth. For that reason, a gastrointestinal (GI) feeding tube was instituted. Only sporadically alert, she was regarded by nurses and Dr. Langston as unable to make her own decisions. As her "attorney-in-fact" (named in her durable power of

attorney for health care, or DPAHC), her husband spoke and
decided for her. He was clearly not happy with this responsibility.

The consulting pulmonologist, Dr. Arthur Richards, emphasized
in a chart note that he regarded continued treatment as "futile,"
because there was nothing he could offer that would provide any benefit. Whatever he could do, he wrote, merely "would prolong her
dying." A do-not-resuscitate, or DNR, order was recommended by
Dr. Langston several days after Dr. Richard's note, but Mr. Oland
insisted at the time, and later, that they must "do everything possible."

Her doctors frequently told him that they had already done
"everything" that could reasonably be done. They in fact told him
that any other treatment, including artificial hydration and nutrition,
was not only not appropriate, but futile. In one conversation documented in the chart, Dr. Langston reported that he had told Mr.
Oland that his wife's living will and power of attorney were now rel-
evant in these circumstances and that she specifically declared in
both that she did not wish to have death "needlessly prolonged."

In the face of Mr. Oland's insistence—"you only get sued by live
people," an intern confided, and several nurses nodded with understanding—full supports continued. Another nephrologist, Dr. Sid
Pennock, agreed with Dr. Langston and thought that Mrs. Oland
would likely not recover sufficiently to be discharged. This, however, was exactly what Mr. Oland said that the family wanted most of
all, even if it meant providing round-the-clock care for her. Dr. Pennock also told Dr. Langston that, in his opinion, Mr. Oland, Janice,
and Charlie were "emotionally unprepared and confused."

In light of their insistence on "doing everything," Dr. Langston
thought that a discussion of clinical ethics would help. I was paged,
given the gist of the situation, and asked to stop by to talk with the
family.

I decided to set up a family conference. I had learned that this family had yet to be together in the same room with the hospital's two
main doctors, Pennock and Langston, and such a meeting was seriously needed. This was a bit difficult to set up, as it had to include
everyone directly involved—the physicians, primary-care nurses,
unit head nurse, hospital chaplain (who had already talked several
times with the family), and the immediate family (it was not possible,
Janice told me, to get her sister to come). I raised the idea with Dr.
Langston, and he asked me to arrange it. I agreed and ended up
moderating.

During our initial discussion, Dr. Langston made it clear that he
had strongly felt for some time there was "something not quite

right" about the Oland family's responses to his talks with them. He wasn't sure just what it was, but he was concerned. He had a sense, he said, that the Oland's were having considerable difficulty confronting something or other. When I pushed him on the matter, he mentioned his impression—"and it's only an impression, you know?"—that when he had earlier discussed the possibility of a feeding tube with Mr. Oland, he had sensed a "sort of strained reaction," especially from Mr. Oland. Janice, Dr. Langston said, seemed "taken aback." The best way he could put it, he said, was that "the atmosphere seemed to change almost tangibly" just at "the moment the GI tube business came up."

Because he didn't think, at the time, that the tube would be an immediate issue, however, he had not pursued the topic then. He nevertheless continued to feel that it might well be the idea of the GI tube that was troubling them. Many people, he said, were troubled by that: "it's just hard for many people to stomach, no pun intended," he concluded. The tube was, in any case, subsequently initiated.

Now that Mrs. Oland's condition warranted serious discussions of removing life supports, he thought the GI tube had probably become "a real hard issue" for them. He warned me to be especially alert to this, since the withdrawal of life supports was an issue that would be extensively discussed at the forthcoming family conference. "And the withdrawal," he lingered over the words, "has to include the feeding tube as well as the ventilator, I hope you understand—I hope they understand!" He assured me that he would himself bring up the matter.

Before setting up the meeting, it was important for me to talk with the Olands myself—immediately, at least to whoever was there at the time. Going to Mrs. Oland's room, I met Mr. Oland and Janice as they were leaving Mrs. Oland's bedside. When I asked Mr. Oland about his son, he told me Charlie had to return home for business reasons but expected to be back tonight or tomorrow morning. Jenny, on the other hand, Janice said forthrightly, "won't be available; she can't stand what's going on."

"Have you talked with her recently?" I asked.

"Oh, yes. I just got off the phone, 'cause one of the nurses, Betty something, said something about a 'family conference' about Momma, and Daddy and I wanted to be sure Jenny knows about that. But . . ."

"Excuse me for butting in," I said, interrupting, "but do you have any idea what is troubling your sister?"

"She's always been awfully close to Momma, and Daddy, too. She's the baby of the family, you know, and just has a really hard time accepting that Momma might not make it. She can't stand to see all these tubes and monitors and such, either. Of course, Charlie and I don't like those things, either, but we know that Momma needs them if she's going to get any better, but," she paused, her voice growing softer, "well, we know Momma's not going to get over this. But Jenny, well, she just falls apart every time anyone mentions that. Anyway, she can't be here; she wants us to just go ahead and do what's right. So it's probably best that she not be here."

Before probing the matter of the feeding tube, I wanted to be much clearer about why they, so Dr. Langston said, kept insisting that "everything be done," especially now that Janice brought it up on her own: "We know that Momma's not going to make it, and it's just so *sad.*"

Which made me wonder, if that's what they think, why were they insisting that she be discharged to her home? Did they know what's really involved in providing these sorts of "supports"—ventilator, suctioning, periodic hemodialysis, not to mention the likely occurrence of fevers and probably even another pneumothorax? Were they aware that Mrs. Oland could hardly go through the trips back and forth to the hospital? Which was just what would happen if they tried to take her home. Or might they instead have been saying something else, maybe that they wanted her to die at home? After all, people do that sort of thing, say one thing and mean something else, especially when it's too awful for them to say out loud, directly. Did they really think it was possible to discharge her, in her "dismal" condition?

So I tried to put at least some of these thoughts into words, as gently as I could: "On another matter, if I may, are you really so sure you want to take your mother back to her home? You know that . . . ," but Janice quickly interrupted me.

"Well, you know, Dr. Zaner," Janice said with surprising candor, "we've known almost from the beginning that Momma's illness, I should say illnesses, were probably just too much for her. And," she went on, "we also know that there is just no way for Daddy to take care of her at home. Heaven knows I can't, not with my job and all, nor Charlie, who has to get back to his family and job, too."

"But haven't you been asking that she be discharged to home?"

"Oh, no," Janice said, looking over at her father, "we've just been . . ."

Then, out of nowhere, Mr. Oland suddenly declared, "Well, *I* surely do, I want her home where she belongs, don't you know, where she's among her things and such."

"Daddy, we've already talked about that . . ."

"You know," I stepped in, "that she's likely to come down with the same sort of problems she already has, and that you'll just have to be taking her back to the hospital time after time."

"That's as may be . . . ," Mr. Oland started out.

But Janice interrupted again. "Daddy, we've talked about this. You know you can't take care of Momma's kidneys and breathing and medicine and such, not as long as she's in need of those treatments, like dialysis. Anyway, Dr. Zaner," she turned to me, clearly the one in charge, "are we supposed to be talking with you about all this?"

"Well, Dr. Langston thought you might want to do just that, though now may not be the best time."

"No time's a good time," Mr. Oland said, looking off down the hallway.

"You know," I said to them before he decided to take off, "that her doctors all think that she's terminal," my so-easy recourse to that worn-out term made me uneasy, but I plunged on, "that she is dying?"

Although I addressed my question directly to Mr. Oland, Janice answered, which made me wonder if her father was in denial or just not paying attention.

"Of course," Janice said. "My goodness, Momma knows, or I should say knew, that, too. That's why she and Daddy both signed those living wills and durable powers of attorney for health care? Charlie and I brought it up, and they were very onto it right away, wanting to sign those things in case one of them or the other got too sick, and they obviously don't want to have things drawn out pointlessly, you know?"

So what, I silently asked myself, was going on here? Was this all just another case of people in the same family not talking or not listening, or what? As we went on, it became clear that Mr. Oland didn't really appreciate what discharge would entail, even though Janice surely did. It was also clear that they realized, on the other hand, that Mrs. Oland was completely bedridden and needed frequent dialysis sessions. Still, Mr. Oland seemed to have only a dim notion of what her dependence on the ventilator, much less the need for suctioning, tube feeding, and so forth implied for taking care of her at home. With Janice objecting, correcting, and insisting, he showed little understanding, for instance, of the fact that her fragile lungs would likely develop additional air leaks, requiring additional chest tubes, meaning likely trips to the operating room, and that even her poor blood pressure could cause serious problems needing prompt medical and nursing attention. If she were at home, she would have to be readmitted many times.

I decided that the apparent disagreement between Janice and her father could get out of hand, especially here in the hallway with others in easy listening distance, without resolving anything of what I had come by to discuss with them. So I pulled the conversation back to that.

"You've indicated that you've heard, of course, about the plan for a family conference. I've arranged for a room, 46R2—it's right down the hall from Mrs. Oland's room—tomorrow morning at 9:00, if that's alright for you. We can set it up at another time."

Janice looked at her father, who nodded, then agreed: "No that's fine; we expect Charlie back tonight. Now, if he can't make it . . ."

"Then we'd just have to reschedule for a time when he will be present," I emphasized, "And, if I may, I know you're anxious to get back to Mrs. Oland, but could I just bring up one other matter?" Janice nodded, but there was no reaction as yet from her father. "Well, I've wondered, Dr. Langston told me just this morning, about the feeding tube . . ."

At this, Mr. Oland looked up sharply, eye to eye for the first time, but before I could go on, he shifted his eyes to Janice, who said, "Yes we know about that, of course, since otherwise Momma can't get any nutrition and water and such."

Mr. Oland, meantime, seemed to shudder. He turned around and seemed ready to walk away, back to his wife's room. "Daddy, wait just a moment, okay? I'm sorry, Dr. Zaner, but Daddy really needs to get back to Momma. Can we talk about all this tomorrow, at the meeting?"

"Of course, that's just what the meeting's for. I hope I haven't upset your father," but Mr. Oland turned back around, his gaze wandering. He looked at me then turned back to his daughter, voice rickety, uncertain. "Myra's waiting, Jannie," he said, "let's go back."

"Mr. Oland, I hope I haven't upset you," I said quickly.

"Dr. whoever . . ."

"Zaner."

"Whatever. I don't know what or who you are, but I'll tell you and anybody else's listening, Myra needs me, bad, especially now that she's so close to being gone. And I got to get back there. Me and Jannie will be there tomorrow for that meeting you say's planned."

And, with that, he turned and again started walking away. Janice grabbed for his arm, though, and stopped him. "Sure," Janice still looking at her father, "tomorrow should be fine. If Charlie's not in tonight, can I call someone and let them know?"

"Here's my numbers, office and home, just let me know, okay? If your brother comes in, though, don't bother calling. I'll just count on seeing you all in the morning?"

"That's fine," she nodded, taking her father's arm and they slowly walked away, back down the hall to Mrs. Oland's room. I was left thinking about Mr. Oland; he seemed so sad, I thought, so awfully sad. And angry. Over what?

I returned to my office on the fourth floor. I couldn't avoid a sense of frustration at myself, mainly because I hadn't gone into the insistent plea that was so disconcerting to Dr. Langston, to "please, do everything" for Mrs. Oland. What do those words mean to Mr. Oland? To Janice? Had Charlie Oland joined them in that insistence? I wondered, too, whether Dr. Langston had perhaps prompted the matter by the way he had discussed her care? For instance, had the feeding tube been initially proposed "so that she can eat and have liquids?"—and, thus, when withdrawal was discussed, did they feel that including the feeding tube would mean that she would "starve to death?" Did Mr. Oland think that his wife, Myra, would die from thirst? Did any of them harbor hidden grudges against the hospital or Dr. Langston? Stan Langston specifically said that both Mrs. Oland's husband and daughter readily acknowledged that she had been given "wonderful" care and were "grateful" that "so very much" had been done for her.

When I had started to talk about the feeding tube, though, Mr. Oland was clearly reluctant; he seemed restrained, even angry, and this puzzled me as much as it had perplexed Dr. Langston. From what I knew of Stan, he was widely regarded as an astute clinician. And, though getting someone to discuss in any depth what that meant—whoever I asked seemed quickly to revert to bad metaphors ("he has a knack . . .")—my own experience with him was much the same: he really was extremely discerning about people.

So, what was going on? Mr. Oland's demeanor bothered me. It seemed as if something were preying on him, as Dr. Langston had suggested, and that he was unable to say anything aloud about it. But what might it be? Did I really sense this, or was I letting myself get carried away by Stan's suggestion and my respect for his clinical discernment? My efforts to get Mr. Oland to talk directly with me had not worked, at least thus far, so at the time I thought it wisest to leave the thing alone until another time and just set up the conference.

Still, the next morning, sitting in the room I'd reserved for the family conference and waiting for everyone to show up, I couldn't help mulling over the situation. Maybe what the Oland's needed was a sense that *they* had "done everything." Discharging Mrs. Oland might mean that *they* would then be directly involved in her care.

Leaving her in the hospital, on the other hand, might mean that they would have left things in the hands of *others*—and that might make them feel they had abandoned her. Hospitals, I knew, not infrequently bring about that sort of feeling, whether welcomed or dreaded. Rather than being "confused," perhaps they were instead in the throes of a kind of anticipatory grief, even guilt. Possibly, they might have been afraid that they would later face that awful sense of "what if . . . ," or "if only we had thought of . . . , then we would have. . . ." While this, too, seemed on track, my thoughts were interrupted by a nurse. I didn't even realize she had come in! In fact, I now realized that the room was rapidly filling. Everyone I had asked to come was there, even Charlie, to whom I introduced myself when I greeted Janice and Mr. Oland. As I began explaining the purpose of the conference, I was hoping the discussion would help ferret out some of these issues.

The two doctors, Langston and Pennock, each in turn carefully reviewed aloud Mrs. Oland's situation from the day of admission. Dr. Langston even included some of his conversations with Dr. Copple, the family physician. Then, I gave each family member a chance to voice any concerns and air questions. It was at once obvious that they did indeed understand that Mrs. Oland was dying, that continuing life supports was merely prolonging her death, and, most important, that discontinuing these supports is precisely what she would want, were she able to talk to us—all of which, indicatively, came out directly in this rather open setting.

It was also clear how much she meant to each of them, how much each needed to be with her and care for her—which may well be the reason they were so focused on trying to persuade the doctors to let them take her home. When I took the chance to ask what their understanding was of that problematic phrase "do everything," Charlie responded. He explained that, by "do everything," they did not in any way think the doctors were holding back anything from his mother or (responding to my own query) that they were centered on their wanting to be involved in her care. Rather, he said, speaking to Dr. Langston, "We've just been so hopeful that you would be able to help Mom get more alert so we could be with her again, even if only one last time."

Janice spoke up, "Yes, Dr. Langston, but also we all want the chance to tell her how much we care, how much we love her, how much she's meant to us."

"And, there's this, too," Charlie said, "Mom could tell us clearly just what she wants done and not done; it would be *her* speaking, her decision. After all, when she came in this time, she really didn't realize she was so bad off, that she's not going to make it. If she had, I'm sure she would have let us know what she thinks."

"Anyway," Janice said softly, "we've got no illusions about her dying and all, and I hope you understand, Dr. Langston, the feeding tube thing hasn't concerned us. We understand about that."

During this exchange, indeed during the entire conference, we heard nothing from Mr. Oland. I noted several times that he was obviously very uncomfortable, nervous, anxious. Something was eating at him. I tried to catch his eye, "Mr. Oland, is this your understanding as well?"

He looked up at me, again with that momentarily sharp-eyed stare I'd seen earlier—which, as suddenly as it had appeared, was gone, though he did manage to say, "That'd be as it may, but we haven't heard from Myra about any of this, now have we? We haven't heard from Myra, and we'd best see to that before anything is done."

"But Mr. Oland," Dr. Langston spoke up quickly, "we've talked about all this many times, you and Myra and me, remember? It was right when you brought her to the hospital and I had done my initial examination. I told you both then that it seemed to me things were not hopeful, and she said she didn't want to be kept on life supports unless she had a good chance of recovering, at least some meaningful degree. Remember?"

Mr. Oland looked thoughtfully at Dr. Langston, then again the sinking down—head, eyes, his whole physiognomy. "As I said, we don't, we can't, we won't do anything 'til Myra has her say," and he just sort of closed in on himself.

Janice and Charlie seemed not a little stunned by their father's outburst, his insistence, in the face of what had just been discussed, acknowledged, agreed to. After a brief silence, Charlie acknowledged that discharge was currently impossible, even though every effort had been made to get her sufficiently able to go home.

Because she had already deteriorated so much, only two options seemed reasonable. (1) Continue current treatments, which I took to mean "indefinitely," that is until she somehow managed to defeat all those efforts and died in spite of them. In this scenario, Mrs. Oland could hang on for perhaps another six months and then would die. More likely, however, she would continue to deteriorate, with multiple infections, additional lung leaks, her nutritional status would diminish, and eventually, within a week or so, she would have a cardiac or pulmonary arrest, or both. Resuscitation, everyone agreed, was not appropriate. Even if she survived the procedure, her death and their grieving would only be prolonged. (2) All life supports should be with-drawn, allowing her to die with as much dignity and comfort as possi-ble in the circumstances.

After much discussion to ensure everyone understood these options, Janice and Charlie—along with the barest of nods from Mr. Oland—agreed to the second proposal. Dialysis would be discontin-ued first, with palliative measures. Dr. Pennock emphasized that Mrs. Oland would experience little if any pain or discomfort. In a few days, he said, she would lapse into a coma, at which point it would then be appropriate to discontinue the ventilator. Soon thereafter, she would die a very peaceful death.

Everyone seemed comfortable with the plan, but the family hoped that they, especially Jenny, would be able to be with Mrs. Oland before she became completely unconscious. She would be moved to a room close to a stairway; that way, family members and friends, even children within the extended family, could enter and leave her room with minimal disturbance to other patients. I knew, as the dis-cussion ended, that there had been far less discussion of the feeding tube than either Stan or I expected. In fact, only Janice and Charlie expressed comfort with its removal. Mr. Oland gave only the barest of nods and seemed disturbed by even that brief discussion.

I left the room even more puzzled: Why did Mr. Oland still appear so dazed yet angry? Was he perhaps disturbed by the tube and, if so, why didn't he tell his children?

Reflecting on the conference, I remained struck by the family's, and the physicians', candor; unusual, it was also highly desirable. Still, at the time, it seemed to me that the lack of reaction by Mr. Oland to the mention of the feeding tube was peculiar. Something was not voiced; it could well be important. So, I decided I had to talk with Mr. Oland again, this time in greater depth and very directly. The next morning I found him in his wife's room and asked him to step outside for a moment; Janice joined us, mentioning that Jenny would be arriving that evening.

"That's good," I said. "But there's something we need to talk about right now; rather, I should say, there seems to me something that you may want to discuss."

"What do you mean?" Janice asked, looking, as she frequently did, at her father. "Daddy? Is there something you haven't told us?"

"Well, I haven't got anything to say that's not already been said by somebody, Jannie. I don't know what you mean," he said, looking pointedly at me. I got the feeling I was on the verge of getting into something which he thought was better left alone, but I sensed I had to plunge ahead, gently but firmly.

"Mr. Oland, when Dr. Langston first asked me to talk with you and your children, he mentioned that he thought you had some sort of reservations, hesitations, like you had something on your mind that you weren't saying out loud. He thought, so he told me, that it might have to do with the feeding tube."

"Why would he think that?" he muttered.

"Why think that?" Janice joined in, "We've said all along that we had no difficulty with it's going in or, now, taking it out. We just hoped that there would be enough time for Momma to be able to be with us some, even a little, before she dies. And that she'll be able to see and talk with Jennie, even her old friend, Abby Dunlop. She's known Abby since they were kids together, and she is trying to get a flight out of Baltimore as we speak. I talked with her this morning."

"Yeah, I know about that, too," Mr. Oland said. "Myra's said to me more than once how much she'd like to see Abby again. It's been some time now, more than five years I think, since they've seen each other. It'd be good," his mood appeared to pick up as he went on, "if they could talk again. Real good. Abbie's a good one, do Myra a world of good. Yes, that'd be dandy . . . ," and his voice trailed off.

He seemed to sink down, as if his body was too heavy. He grew smaller. As Janice and I continued, he gave no sign of hearing us. I again mentioned how Dr. Langston was also worried, at which point Mr. Oland came back up, if only slightly, from that pit in which he had sunk since we first talked.

"Dr. Langston just shouldn't say things like that," he suddenly exploded.

"Like what?" I asked, surprised.

"Well," he paused, wavering on the edge of something. Then he appeared to come to a decision, "You know, things like, that Myra's just doing no good and, well, . . ."

Again he broke off, unable to go on. Janice and I sat quietly, waiting. Mr. Oland glanced at Janice, but her eyes were averted, filled with tears as she felt her father's grief and sadness.

"It just seems to me," he said, eyes downcast, "that you shouldn't say, just right out like that, that, that, Myra wouldn't want us to help, to get her better so we can get her back home." Though still suffering, his voice grew increasingly assertive. "I *know* what the doctors and others said in that conference yesterday. But it's just so *unfair*, you know? *Home*, that's where she belongs. *That's* where she *belongs*, and where she *wants* to be. *Dammit*, she just don't want to be in this damned hospital. We *got* to get her out of here and back home. Now you listen to me, young man, you got to tell that doctor that Myra's got to be done *right*, taken home, and I just don't care what he says."

Janice seemed stung when he blurted out "*dammit.*" She looked at him murmuring, "Oh, Daddy, don't, just don't." Looking at me, she said, "Please, you've got to understand. Daddy is just so upset, wants Momma home so much, he . . ."

"Jannie," Mr. Oland broke in, "just hush, right now. It's about time I had my own say for myself. You *know* Mamma don't like this place, don't like it at all. You *know* that, and you know we've just *got* to get her back *home* where she belongs, and if it means it's just to die, well then okay, but home's the place it oughta be. It just isn't *right* to make us leave her here, what with all that damned stuff they got her hooked up to, and her barely breathing and struggling so much, my God, that isn't right, not right at all. I already talked to her, and she told me so . . ."

"You already discussed this with her?" I said, "But you haven't mentioned this before. Are you sure?" I knew I shouldn't have put it that way, but this came as a real surprise, especially in light of what Stan had told me more than once.

"Well," again he had difficulty getting his thoughts into words. "Well, yeah, in a way."

"Please, Mr. Oland, go on. What is it you talked about?"

"Well, you know, before she began to fade here a month or so ago," his speech was wooden, then slowly picked up again, "but that isn't the point anyway, by damn! I just *know* what Myra'd want and not want, and she wants to go *home*. Besides, I'm her whatchamacallit, aren't I? Her . . ."

"Her attorney-in-fact," I said for him.

"Yeah, that, and what I say goes, isn't that right?"

"I know, Daddy. I know," Janice sobbed softly.

Because he seemed so disturbed, I wondered whether it would be better to wait for another occasion before revisiting whatever it was that was bothering him. I was still unsure, maybe something about that feeding tube. So, I suggested that we continue this conversation later. Janice quickly agreed, taking his arm and helping him into Mrs. Oland's room. But before I could leave, she turned back, and drew me aside. "You've got to understand, Dr. Zaner. Daddy is just not himself. All that language, it's just not like him. He's not an angry person, never has been. And he's usually not so reticent. I just don't understand."

"He certainly does seem rather disturbed and angry."

"But that's just the point, you see, he's not an *angry* man, that's just not his way at all. He's a sweet, gentle man. He *never* uses words like that, never talks to people that way. I *know* something's wrong, that he's really bothered about something; otherwise he wouldn't act that way. I thought we had talked it all out, that he understood, especially after that conference. Not just that Mamma isn't going to make it, but that we just can't take her home. I *know* he knows."

"What do you think is on his mind, then?"

She went on to say that he really was terribly disturbed about something, but she didn't know what it might be. But, she emphasized that when she had talked with him even before I had first met with them, he seemed increasingly closed up. He wouldn't really talk to her, not the way he most often did, and when she asked several times what was bothering him, he just clammed up, sank down, became sort of not there. She thought that during the conference he'd gotten whatever it was that was bothering him under control. He was more like his "real self" then, at least until I cornered him afterward.

"But when we talked after the meeting, well, that's just not like him. We've always been able to talk about the most difficult things. Now," she hesitated, trying to find the words. "Now, I just know that something's wrong."

"Don't you think it's important to find out what it is? It's not going to help if he stays angry and upset."

"But, I don't think he's angry, you see?

"I'm sorry, I didn't mean 'angry,' but he does seem quite upset. What's going on? Do you have any idea?"

"Well, I'm not sure, but I know what you mean, about the importance of finding out and all. There's something festering inside him, and he won't admit it, won't talk about it at all. Can you help?"

"I'm not at all sure," I said, " Let me be candid: are any of you worried about the feeding tube? That's something that wasn't addressed very directly in the meeting, and it occurred to Dr. Langston that it might be what's bothering your father. You know, the newspapers and TV have been filled with the discussions about assisted suicide, euthanasia, and that sort of thing—what with Kevorkian and all these court cases."

"Feeding tube?" she asked, surprise all over her voice and face. "What do you mean? Isn't that just one of those 'life supports' that aren't going to be kept up now? Why would we worry about that?"

"You're *not?*"

"Not at all."

"But what about your father? When we first talked and I mentioned the tube, he seemed to me very restrained, as if . . ."

"No, I don't think so. We all talked about all that yesterday before the conference, and, no, I don't think any of us is concerned about that."

"Did you all actually discuss it?" Anxiety was getting the best of me, but I pressed on "Some people seem to think that pulling the feeding tube is the same thing as starving a person. And though, from everything I know, that is not an appropriate concern, it is terribly symbolic."

"We know all that, Dr. Zaner, but, really, that hasn't bothered us."

So much for Stan's and my suspicions. What, then, was behind Mr. Oland's behavior? What was going on here?

After leaving them, I went down to the cafeteria. Time for some strong coffee. It was clear to me that something else was bothering him. Janice noted it, too, had seen it for some time now.

I wasn't sure how to get to it, but another conversation seemed in order. I stopped by the next day, and, sure enough, Mr. Oland was there. Janice, however, was not. "She's gone to pick up Jenny," Mr. Oland said, "'cause Jenny couldn't get here last night, had to take a later plane that only just arrived." He looked at his watch.

"Could we talk for a moment, Mr. Oland? There's something still bothering me from yesterday."

"I suppose so, if you must." Willing, but reluctant. We went back into the conference room. With considerable courage, he was able to dredge up the thing that had so preyed on him.

"I get the impression, Mr. Oland, that something is really eating at you, and others have noticed the same thing—Janice, Dr. Langston, even Betty Joseph, your wife's main nurse, spoke to me about this."

"Well, I'm not at all sure what you're talking about, young man." Which amused me, I am hardly 'young' any more. But I could tell he was already backing into that damnable pit, that inability or unwillingness to talk. So I jumped in. "I'm not all that 'young,' you know?" I said, "After all, my daughter is almost at middle age, my son not far behind."

"No kidding?" he bobbed back up again and into our conversation. "How old's your daughter? And what's she do anyway?"

"Well, I'm not sure I should be letting out her age—she's certain to get a bit upset, right? Anyway, she surprised everyone, becoming a real, grade-A computer expert: she works in the research division at Microsoft. Imagine, my daughter a corporate person despite her father and mother!"

"Well, now, that seems just real fine, real nice, knowing all about computers and such."

"It is, to be sure; I don't mean to knock it at all. More, though, she's happy with what she's doing."

"That's wonderful; I guess you're real proud, aren't you?"

"To say the least. And you must be very proud of your children, too, I bet. But, I've gotten off what I wanted to discuss with you. Forgive me if I'm a bit blunt, but I do think this is important, for you and your family: is there something you've not mentioned, not to your family or to anyone else? Something that's really hard to talk about?"

He slumped back in the chair. His eyes dropped, his face sagged, his lips bubbled ever so slightly, his hands anxious. Then, he sat up, obviously disturbed, as he told his story.

Somehow he had managed to get it in his mind that *he* was to blame for the crisis that led to his wife's being hospitalized. While he knew that she had "problems," as he put it, for a long time, she remained active. "Hell, she even played a little golf up until we had to bring her in here." He said he never really tried to persuade her to go more slowly. "She just needed, you know, well, to take it easier. 'Course, this is now, that then was then. I just didn't say much at the time, and I should have . . . ," and his voice trailed off.

And there it was, or there some of it was: a bitter sense of guilt, a fault he found in himself. Still, there was more to it. Beneath that increasingly corrosive sense of guilt, an even more vexing difficulty gradually emerged. In a way, he recognized that blaming himself over not being more persistent in getting her to ease off just didn't ring completely true.

"Naw, that's not it, I know it wasn't no fault of mine. Myra's been strong headed all her life, don't I know! But it was just so hard to talk, there toward the time when I brought her here. So damned hard!"

"I think I understand, Mr. Oland," I said, "but you did have some talk, didn't you? Like when you realized she needed to be here?"

"Myra's known about her problems—that she's been awfully sick 'n all—and was worried over what might likely happen if she was put in the hospital. More'n once she had tried to talk about the matter—especially about her maybe not making it . . ."

He grew silent, then, very softly he spoke again. "She really did try to talk about all this," which I gathered meant precisely what in fact happened: "All those tubes and things," as he'd said earlier. But then, again, his voice dropped to little more than a whisper. As I listened, as I began to understand what had been going on with him, his demeanor made sense.

He simply *could not* talk about that, about death, about her death, with Myra, so he had taken to walking out whenever she started in on the matter. He couldn't talk about it because that meant he'd have to face losing her and couldn't bear even the merest inkling about that, not Myra, his dear, sweet Myra whom he'd known for so long.

Nor could he face the dreadful prospect of sitting day after day in the waiting room. "How the hell can I do that," he jabbed out the words, "I'd see her so little, be with her so little and, with all those damned tubes and drugs and such, she'd be out of it most of the time, and that I can't bear, just can't bear it, not at all, never, and most of all living alone in that house, empty, hollowed out, it seems, without her but with all her things, Myra herself, right there in that bed, that sheet, that clothes closet, even those shoes she's always complaining about but won't get rid of—awful, all of them, but they are *her*, everything in that house is her, all of it, can't stand even to make myself a cup of coffee, and how can I go on living with them all around all the time?"

Which, sadly, is just what happened, and now he simply couldn't, as he said, bear it. And which, too, was why he'd been trying so hard to get Stan to release her to go home, home where at least she would be there among her things, be herself, and that could let him be himself again, maybe, somehow, some way, couldn't I see?

Racked with guilt that he had failed her, his life's only partner, he now felt himself an utter failure. Coupled with that, though, there gradually emerged a still harsher, though veiled, sense of profound remorse: *he hadn't even let her talk, not even when she'd wanted to talk*, about what she wanted the doctors to do, nor even about her all but certain death. Then, when they had asked him, as her decision maker at that time, if he knew what she wanted done, he was stunned into silence. *He didn't know*, because he hadn't wanted her to talk, hadn't let her talk, about any of that, and she had eventually stopped trying. *But of course, he did know, he knew his* Myra, *didn't he, after all these years together?* He couldn't face any of it—that he'd not let her talk with him, nor him with her, nor let himself even think about that awful prospect, nor bring himself even to think about those awful things.

Later, after Mrs. Oland's dialysis was discontinued with the expectation that she would soon lapse into a final coma, she surprisingly became more alert. Her family could be with her, at least for a time, and discussions previously impossible were now imperative: What did she say about being terminally ill? What was going on with Mr. Oland?

As I went into her room one evening, she wasn't the least surprised to see me, not even when I introduced myself as an "ethicist." Though still intubated, she responded to my questions with her eyes, through nods and hand gestures. She was in fact one of the most expressive people I've known, and I got a hint, a slight clue, of the woman she must have been, and with that a new appreciation of what Mr. Oland had been going through all these weeks: could I have done any better were it my own precious wife in that condition?

Apparently more alert than any of us realized, she indicated, not without a chuckle, that she was quite clear about her wishes, was bothered by all the attention, and obviously didn't want any more of it. Having led a rewarding life, she was ready for whatever would now transpire and did not want life supports continued. She did want the chance to be with her family a last time and was grateful to learn she had been transferred to another room that would permit them to come and go at will. She wanted to see her old friend, Abby Dunlop. She was anxious to talk with her husband; she knew how terribly he had suffered. I stepped out of the room, to find him.

Betty, her nurse, later told me that the very evening after I talked with her, a party took place in her room, which was crowded with relatives. Mrs. Oland was even able to indulge a can of cold beer through the feeding tube! Her son later told me that everyone was deeply moved, especially his mother, by the conversations over the past several days. All that remained, he said, was for her to see her best friend, but they were worried that this might prove impossible, because her flight had already been cancelled once. In fact, it might take several days before Abby Dunlop could get to the hospital. Dr. Langston assured him that he would do everything he could to ensure that she would remain alert until Abby arrived.

As it turned out, though, he didn't have to do much. Mrs. Oland managed to stay alert for the next two days. Abby Dunlop came, and they visited for several hours. After, Mrs. Oland was at peace. She gradually slipped deeper into a coma and died several days later.

I need to map, even if only initially, some prominences on the landscape of my encounter with the Oland family, both for its own sake and for the sake of other sick people I meet every day.

There she was, lying on the bed, very still, quiet, seemingly, deceptively, at peace with herself and the world, the ventilator's chug and the faint whoosh of the air conditioning the only sounds. Her eyes flickered, then opened, partially and irregularly, without apparent stimulus. When I said her name, her head turned toward me, or my voice. But, though her eyes opened, they were unfocused, wandering, unseeing. I spoke again, gave my name and mentioning that I was from clinical ethics, that her doctor asked me to stop by. She didn't seem to orient to me; it seemed that she did not hear me (a mistake, I later learned, though understandable). I said goodbye and quietly left.

Much later, after she regained alertness, things were markedly different. When I entered her room this time, she turned her head, looked at me, and, despite the tubes and lines hooked up to her body, was very much a lively, vivid presence.[2] She nodded when I spoke, her eyes wrinkled with humor, she even managed to smile around the ventilator tube. She raised her hands from time to time, displaying or emphasizing her feelings, which she also managed to express physiognomically, with her eyes, eyebrows, face, hands.[3] She was animated, spry.

When I said my name, her eyes glittered with recognition. As surprise shot across my face, her eyes crinkled and her cheeks seemed almost aglow with obvious amusement—this lady did enjoy being playful. She had heard me in my earlier visit, it was clear. Later in this conversation, while talking about her condition quick impatience was followed by gestured understanding. Mention of her husband's difficulties brought tears, averted eyes, a slow raising, turning over, and dropping of her hand: great sadness, regret. My discomfort was evident to me; so was it to her, despite her despondency. We were vividly present to each other.

In Alfred Schutz's lovely phrase, she and I were face-to-face with each other, making music together: she within her own history and still-unfolding biography, me within mine. At first, though, this mutual presence seemed more a sort of promise, one that might or might not be fulfilled, depending on what transpired between us. But, because she was terminally ill and I would soon be on my way elsewhere, this clearly remained a mere promise of what could have been. However minimal and temporary, this encounter was deeply textured with our biographies, our lives. Our meeting was dense with anecdotes and tales, their themes embedded in stories that were invited (and could, even might have been elaborated) in every glance and gesture. There was here the promise of sharing that, since impossible, was equally redolent with sadness, a recognition of limitation, borders with sharp edges.

If I had met her on the street, merely looking and being looked at as we passed by a department store, this too would have been an incipient invitation to participate in each other's biographies and histories—though nowhere as intense as being in her hospital room. Even with her being "out of it," or so I thought on our first meeting, I found myself within a rich context of potential dialogue, talking and listening, and wondered: can she hear me? When we met I entered her history and found her a part of my own. For all the boundaries and limits, the "mere" promise of a future, there was a kind of "we."

To enter *the* room was to enter *her* room. I noticed straightaway that, even if she didn't orient to me, everything in the room, including me, was *oriented to her* in very specific and powerful ways. *She* was the center; everything in the room was there for *her;* she was the focus for all the equipment, activity, procedures, and anyone who came in (nurses, doctors, family, visitors). Talk, too, centered on her, had to do with her (even while the "same" room would, of course, be used later by others, who would then also be a centering presence). Though unable to talk at first, what talk there was among those in her room, even small talk, was geared to or, most often, *about* her. Doctors' and nurses' talk swung attention to her: What was going on? What went wrong? How long will she be this way? What can be expected to happen next? Is there anything we can do?

Not only words, but even gestures, tended to be muted in her presence, as if being able to wander around or shake hands was intrusive, even insulting—an unwelcome reminder of things once within her repertoire but now no longer. This was especially true of Mrs. Oland, who couldn't even sit up or, because of intubation, talk, much less walk about. I felt real discomfort, awkwardness, in being able to do all that when she could not, a sense that was not completely dispelled when she later tried to put me at ease.

I noted that, despite her vulnerability—more accurately, *because* of it—she was compelling, a commanding presence simply by being there, in that room, in that hospital. She was the centering place and occasion with respect to which everything was organized and arranged—furniture, equipment, people, professionals, television. This contrasted strikingly with the social-structural imbalances due to her illness and her relationship with others of us, but especially her doctors—with those who were able to do what she could not: if she wanted a sip of water, others had to act; if she needed bedsores attended, the nurse had to act; if she needed drugs for pain, the doctor had to act. Her relationship to the rest of us was asymmetrical, especially to doctors and nurses, with power on their side, not hers; they knew, she didn't; they could, she couldn't.

Dr. Langston, her attending, had the knowledge and skills necessary for diagnosing and treating her; she did not. He, not she, had access to resources (diagnostic technologies, equipment, prescription drugs, consultants, hospitals). Moreover, Dr. Langston and others like him were legally authorized and socially legitimated to use their knowledge, access, and skills on *her*, the very one who was sick and debilitated, the one who knew and understood least of all. Her vulnerability was striking. Not only was she compromised by her condition, but she was also disadvantaged by that very relationship.[4]

The illness experience is unique, just as are the specific efforts to "do something" about an illness. Intrusive and unwanted, illness seems a capricious irruption of our ongoing lives, marked by a sense of urgency and underlain by the threat of compromise and loss (time, ability, funds, family, friends), and ultimately of death. Mrs. Oland's illness cut into the fabric of her social, familial, and individual life, abruptly altering her usual relations with other people—especially Mr. Oland—and severely compromising her sense of herself and her world.

She had to contend with the various crises brought on by illness just at a time when she did not know what was going on, what could and should be done about it, or just what to expect. Her energy was utterly absorbed and focused by trauma, pain, shock, regret, loss, distress. Most likely, not only did she not know Dr. Langston (like she knew her own doctor), but she didn't even know whether he could in fact help her—even though his very presence in the hospital (and all that includes) itself professed that he had the ability to help, heal, or cure.

Despite his, or any physician's, claims of competence and trustworthiness, she had no direct knowledge or experience that could possibly serve to warrant her initial act of trust in him.[5] She, like most of us, may have tried to ignore her illness, or to rely on her own resources—a dietary regimen of vitamins and minerals. Except for that, however, help from someone else had to be sought. She thereby entered into that structurally asymmetrical relationship powerfully reinforced by the institution, the hospital itself.

It was perfectly evident: the physician, not the patient and not the family, had the advantage over this terribly vulnerable elderly woman and her family. The asymmetry was not merely a formality of social structure but an existential reality, a vital fact of life, especially in this hospital and in these circumstances. As one patient poignantly remarked, "You have to trust these people, the physicians, like you do God. You're all in their hands, and if they don't take care of you, who's going to?" Doctors are "overpowering," another emphasized. "They've got an edge on you."

In these plaintive words is the echo of an ancient enigma I've had many occasions to think about, and certainly it is one I encountered every moment I was involved with the Olands. The sense of it is unmistakable even if difficult, even embarrassing to admit openly: the multiple temptations implicit to having real power over a person who is sick and therefore wholly vulnerable and exposed (to gazes, touches, voices, not to mention the far more intrusive interventions common to many medical encounters). The puzzle is at the very heart of the typical, much-acclaimed relationship between patients and physicians. It is indeed the nub of the Hippocratic tradition, especially challenging in the mythic sources of the oath. The medical historian Ludwig Edelstein saw the essential point: "What about the patient who is putting himself and 'his all' into the hands of the physician?"[6] Is the patient's initial trust in a physician warranted?

At the wellspring of the tradition is the god Apollo and his progeny Asclepius, the god of both healers and patients. Physicians who took the oath understood that they were thereby pledged to help all sick and injured people, without prejudice. They understood that the "art" (*techne*) of medicine unavoidably involved them with sick people and their families in potent and uniquely intimate ways, at times called on to render judgments and make decisions that reached far beyond the application of merely technical knowledge and skills. These ancient healers believed they were entrusted by the gods with a supreme wisdom about afflicted people; their vow committed them to be as attentive to the soul as they had to be to the body. Indeed, they thought that the soul could be affected only through the body.

The Asclepian healing places were open to every sick or injured person, whether the person was slave or free, pauper or prince, man or woman. Following the guidance of Asclepius, for whom the virtue of philanthropy was paramount, the healer thereby took on certain fundamental responsibilities. First and foremost, it was said, would-be healers had to turn their attention to themselves, to heal themselves first, before ever trying to serve others. Thus, in addition to justice and self-restraint, the healer had to have the courage to deliberate on and heal himself before attempting to heal the sick.

Behind the covenant to Asclepius, and his daughters Hygieia and Panaceia, is an understanding of social life—in particular, that form thanks to which a vulnerable sick person would at all think about entering into a face-to-face but asymmetric relationship with a

professed healer and the considerable powers of the art. The
covenant thus sworn to invokes a moral vision centered on the
healer-patient relationship—wherein power speaks to vulnerability,
the one who has power over against the one made vulnerable by sickness. This oath thus shows a strong sense of the power inherent in
the art, its seductive potential for control, influence and even vio-
lence to the patient and family who come to be "in the hands" of a
healer. Acting on behalf of the sick person and maintaining strict
silence about all things learned from the relationship were as integral
to the oath as were certain conducts strictly banned (giving aborti-
facents, assisting a suicide, performing a lithotomy).

Incorporating that blend of virtues (justice or fairness, disciplined
self-restraint, and courage), the ancient practitioner of the art thus
clearly recognized his unique position to take advantage of people at
that very time in their lives, on the other hand, when they are especially vulnerable and accessible. The oath also strongly suggests a
recognition of the central challenge and temptation inherent to the
work of the physician; the oath is among the earliest stages in the
emergence of a sophisticated moral cognizance.

This striking moral cognizance is also puzzling. It forces a search-
ing moral question: What could possibly prompt a healer *not* to take
advantage of a vulnerable patient? Why not take advantage precisely
because the patient is vulnerable and cannot get back at you? Just
here, buried squarely within the Hippocratic tradition, is that ancient
puzzle. Another equally ancient and powerful myth about the temptation of having actual power gives needed perspective: the Gyges
story in book 2 of Plato's *Republic*—a scene that postulates a very different kind of social life than that in the Hippocratic tradition.

The theme is justice and injustice. Thrasymachus, a notable
Sophist, advances the idea that injustice is more powerful than justice. In fact, he argues, justice is a sham. Given the chance, people
will pursue whatever is to their own advantage. Even in a system
ruled by law, people comply with the law only against their native
inclinations—whether from fear of retribution, indolence, or simply
because they lack the power to do as they wish. Granted the freedom
to act, both those who are "just" and those who are "unjust" will be
caught red-handed doing the same thing, pursuing their own personal advantage.

Socrates has us imagine someone with the power possessed by the
fabled Gyges, a shepherd in the service of the ruler of Lydia. An
earthquake had opened up a deep chasm. When he went down into
the crevice, Gyges found a hollow bronze horse inside which was a

human corpse wearing nothing but a gold ring. Without detectable
reflection, he (like most of us, one supposes) promptly removed the
ring and placed it on his own finger. During a meeting with other
shepherds, he chanced to twist the ring's collet to the inside and
promptly became invisible, without, apparently, the others noticing.
Marveling at this, he turned the collet the other way and—presto!—
reappeared, again without the others apparently noticing that he'd
been "gone." Gyges' response is well known: he managed to have
himself appointed as one of the monthly messengers to the king. On
his arrival, he turned the ring's collet, then seduced the queen, and
with her help killed the king and took the crown for himself.

   With such a ring and having no fear of capture, both the "just" and
"unjust" will act the same way: that each seeks to gain the advantage
over the other is the governing norm; "just" and "unjust" are but social
conventions, merely words. The question is *not* how the ring's power
should be used; morality is merely the invention of those who can
enforce their wishes. The only questions are *who* now has the power
and how the power *will* be used, for it most assuredly will be used.

   In this framework, the enigma buried within the Hippocratic tradition and its oath can be dramatically displayed: after all, isn't the
Gygean idea about the nature of human and social life really correct?
Isn't each of us out for our own self-interest? Having the advantage,
thanks to the "ring's" power, a Gygean healer will obviously take
advantage of those who are vulnerable *precisely because* they are vulnerable, openly accessible for seduction or being overpowered (as
were the queen and king of Lydia). More's the marvel, none would
even suspect what had happened. Such is the "ring's" true power, to
be capable of use without detection. If the Gygean vision of sociality
is true, the healing art must perforce be interpreted from that stand-
point, and that makes the oath a clever fraud, a guise for the exercise
of power, of whatever sort it may be. Anything else is façade; the truth
of human life is power, vulnerability merely motive for its exercise.

   When people are strangers to each other, with little or no knowledge of their respective beliefs, conducts, values, and the like, there is
obviously all the more reason for suspicion and distrust as the basic
form of social life. The Gygean myth strikes home: when the grounds
for trust within a helping relation are missing, or at the very least are
quite problematic, we would all act, as Thrasymachus might have said,
like Gyges. The relationship between healer and patient is constituted
by the asymmetry of power in favor of the healer over against the vulnerability of the one seeking the healer's help. Although concealed
within social conventions of bedside manner (politeness, courtesy,

civility, and the like), as Hobbes postulated in his *Leviathan*, beneath it all is the self-seeking of Gyges and the ring of power.

To begin with the social construction implicit to the Gyges myth, or Hobbesian leviathan, however, makes fraudulent nonsense of the Asclepian-Hippocratic understanding of the art of medicine and the relationship with sick and injured people. Even so, to accept the popular postulate of self-interest as the basis of human social relations is ineluctably to pose the fundamental question. If the healer is to be entrusted with such power and intimacies (affecting the body, the person, the family, the household, and, more broadly, the social sphere), the crucial question concerns what the healer must do and be to earn, ensure and preserve that trust (i.e., to be trustworthy within a social matrix that makes of trust a mere disguise for the use of power).

Why *not* use the asymmetry of the relationship, much less the vulnerability of illness, for the healer's own advantage? Whoever possesses the ring will surely use it to further his or her own self-interest. The one who seeks the healer's help, however, has little choice but to trust precisely while being at the mercy of the healer, the very one who professes and then proceeds to use the power of the art (knowledge, skills, resources), who proposes and then proceeds to engage in highly intimate, potent, and consequential actions on people who are at their most vulnerable. Illness, injury, and human affliction more generally—among the few authentic universals in human life—give the lie to the Gygean vision of social life.

Each myth invokes its own vision of the social world, including clinical encounters. In both, one with power and advantage confronts another who is relatively powerless and at a decided disadvantage. In the Hippocratic tradition, the potencies of the art were clearly appreciated and given expression in its oath, specifically in its repeated injunctions: to act always *on behalf of* the sick person, never to take advantage of the patient or his family or household (for instance have sexual relations), never to "spread abroad" what is learned in the privacy of the relationship with the sick person, and so forth. In the Gyges tale, to the contrary, the therapeutic act can make no sense: why engage in healing, since that will only allow the vulnerable to become less vulnerable? But if therapy must be read as Asclepian, we still face the grave moral issue, one that has been an abiding part of medicine's history: why "act in the patient's interest," much less "do no harm?"

The clinical event is a very special sort of relationship, for it is inherently haunted by Gyges: the extraordinary temptation to manipulate, control, or otherwise take advantage of the ineluctably vulnerable person. Why Asclepius and not Gyges? It may be that it is in the mythic interplay between these images that the moral character of encountering the other-as-ill is best understood.

This mythic interplay provides a fascinating opening for probing the puzzle at the heart of any clinical encounter. The Hippocratic tradition sets forth, Edelstein points out, a "morality of the highest order." No matter how you look at it, such a life must seem wholly unlivable, its virtues unachievable, its "sacred" character unfeasible at best, and thus medicine a thoroughly impractical practice—unless read as a pretext for Gyges, a reading not altogether unfamiliar to us: physicians, enjoying unprecedented prestige and social power and seeking to enhance them. In other words, while the ancient art seems unable to abide a Gygean reading, a Gyges may nevertheless nestle snugly within each of us; it surely haunts the clinical relationship.

Yet, there was something peculiar, even paradoxical, about Mrs. Oland's vulnerability, and about those immediately affected, such as Mr. Oland or Janice. Precisely because she was so vulnerable, Mrs. Oland, like most patients, was *compelling*. Whether ill, injured, or crippled by genetic or congenital accident, simply by lying there bedridden and unable to help herself, she drew our attention; she was magnetic. It was almost as if in that very presentation she was a center of gravity pulling others' looks, gestures, and words toward her. Walking into her room, I sensed that I really should do or have done or said something, but I felt as if the mere act of walking in and looking around were itself a sort of trespass onto forbidden terrain. Yet I wanted to be understanding and helpful. In this sense, compassion seems ready to hand even if it is not always clear just how it should be realized in each particular situation. Thus, while I wanted to be helpful, I was never quite sure just what that meant in the here and now.

I was aware that her compelling magnetism emerged mainly because, standing there, I inevitably experienced the significant *differences* between us—her illness contrasted with my wellness, her *vulnerability* with my ability to do what she could not. And I found myself contrasting that with the vibrancy that is so obvious in those who, like Janet or some other visitor, are well: the look of the eyes (welcoming, threatening), the lift of flesh (gladness, dismay), speaking (irony, seriousness). It was just this muting of aliveness characteristic of illness, its very silence, that made her all the more prominent and exposed.

In particular, Mrs. Oland's body had a kind of pallor and wanness that of itself provoked moral cognizance, as Hans Jonas observed,[7] even prompting one to wonder whether she was still a vibrant presence within that embodying form. This was immediately evident when I first went in to see Mrs. Oland: gowned and flat on her back in bed, utterly reliant on mostly anonymous others, equipment hooked up to her failing body, and her apparent but fruitless efforts to focus. It was also apparent when I met her on the second occasion, though there were obvious differences: her eyes, hands, even facial color had become more lively; they spoke and, in this, they bespoke her presence.

To be sure, her very vulnerability (especially when she was not alert) left her open to the actions (nurturing or otherwise) of other people; to medical and nursing examinations, for instance. Yet, that very exposure was morally commanding and compelling. I sensed it immediately on entering her room: *Don't touch anything! Watch what you say!* I noted how potent was that vulnerability; it attracted, directed anyone who approached to be careful in what was said and done. I sensed that I was silently governed by a need to be restrained yet concerned, just because she was so sick, so vulnerable. It would be monstrous to take advantage of her. Not that she could not be manipulated, although the condition for that to occur may well be an ability to ignore her presence as person.

That very presence as vulnerable of itself evokes a moral cognizance, as both Albert Schweitzer[8] and Herbert Spiegelberg understood.[9] The very imbalance of the helper/person-helped relationship was, paradoxically, turned on its head. This elemental moral alertness suggests a primary sense of responsibility.[10] Buried within this experience, that alertness was first articulated by ancient physicians at least as early as the Hippocratic Oath. Indeed, the oath's strong insistence on justice and self-restraint (and, I believe, courage) is remarkable, for that very relationship places power on the side of the physician, not the patient.

Mrs. Oland was multiply disadvantaged: by her illness, her separation from familiar activities and people and things, her relative lack of knowledge of her condition, her unavoidable focus on pain and her failed and failing bodily abilities, but also by the very relationship with her would-be healers, Drs. Langston and Pennock, not to mention others of us who entered her domain, even with the intent of helping. The responsibility—*never take advantage of the patient*—has its source in that awesome vulnerability and, as Edelstein notes many times, constitutes the heart of the physician's professional duties. Nothing—we must interpret this stringency—can be allowed to take precedence over that responsibility.

Spiegelberg notes that this is not so much a "principle" as it is an appeal to each of us to undergo the awakening of "a moral sense that is usually dormant but that on special occasions can be brought to the surface."[11] Grievous illness is just such an occasion. Walking into Mrs. Oland's room, I found myself feeling that very awakening, a sense of being called on or of finding myself in the immediacy of her compelling need and my will to help her, to do something for her, this specific unique person, perchance to ease her pain and assuage her suffering, but at the very least to ease and comfort her with whatever it is I may have: words, touches, looks.

The ability any doctor possesses to alter a patient's life has different aspects. It is, for instance, a *power for* (acting on her behalf as she defines it, regardless of whether I agree); it is also a *power over* (paternalism, acting on her behalf as I define it, ignoring her wishes) and even a *power with* (shared decisions, mutual trust, acting on her behalf as we have worked it out over the course of time and shared concern). In each case, however, and whether one or another interpretation of the structural imbalance of the relationship is appropriate or correct in any situation, the power (as the ability to effect changes) has as its focus the vulnerable sick person. Although its focus on healing and helping makes medicine an inherently moral enterprise, this more specifically emerges from the asymmetry of the clinical event—its display of the beguiling possibility of seduction, of taking advantage of persons whose lives are in the nature of the case precarious and compellingly exposed. Precisely because the physician can take advantage, therefore this ought never be done.

Alfred Schutz has vividly demonstrated that in our daily lives, we for the most part live, act, and think within a more or less thoroughly taken-for-granted context of relatively well-defined typifications—of types of people, sorts of things and relations, kinds of activities. So long as our affairs remain relatively settled and unruffled, for the most part we simply take for granted certain key expectations and assumptions, "idealizations," as he calls them.[12] Our typical and typifying ways of thinking and acting together in the everyday world are maintained so long as nothing comes along to upset or unsettle them. They remain "valid" for the most part and for all practical purposes—in particular our taken-for-granted and typified expectations that partners in social action share pretty much the same practical purposes and assumptions.

Just an unsettling of taken-for-granted presumptions is at the heart of encounters between strangers, because the stranger is essentially one who has no choice but to wonder about and even question nearly everything that is taken for granted by the people approached. With this in mind, it is clear that neither the Olands nor I participated in one another's prior and ongoing lives and histories outside the context of the hospital and Mrs. Oland's illness. From their (or my) perspective they (or I) were strangers. Indeed, the stranger, Schutz emphasizes, is one without a shared history.[13] The stranger knows *that* the group whose "home" he is seeking entry to has its own folkways and mores and thus also knows that these are not an integral part of his own biography. From the perspective of those "at home," on the other hand, although the stranger is seen as having *a* culture and history, even a personal biography, these are precisely what is not known (or known only barely, in mere outline, as typified). Hence, those at home cannot take for granted regarding the stranger what they otherwise typically take for granted regarding each other.

The familiar and the routine, the settled and the comfortable, including the common tongue, are now no longer able to be taken for granted by the stranger. Rather than proceeding on the presumption of shared values and outlooks, conversations with the stranger assume the form of probings and explorations. Thus, they are always problematic and textured by uncertainties.

Yet conversations (verbal and nonverbal) are the only means by which strangeness can be overcome and the grounds for trust, even though temporary, established. It is one thing to urge that trust requires meaningful conversation between physician and patient. It is quite another to understand what conversation must be to encourage, or even allow for, trust. What does "talk" have to do with "trust?"

It was already well recognized by ancient Hippocratic healers that the one who professes to heal must be a "physician of the soul as well as of the body" and should "heal thyself" before undertaking relationships with patients. A key part of that relationship is *talk:* asking, listening, and so on, exhibiting some of the features of dialogue. In any dialogue, there is a vulnerability that marks out the existential situation of the questioner, the one who openly admits to a form of vital not knowing or inability to know. In working on this premise, the Socratic dialogical mode verges closely on what seems significant about clinical encounters, even while the phenomenon of special vulnerability surely differs. In the one, the spiritual need is great but the person is presumably healthy, enough at least to carry on the dialogue. In the other, however, the very fact of illness (patient) or distress (family) itself compromises both spiritual and bodily abilities; thus, too, language, plain talking and listening. The vulnerability presented by sickness or distress, whether the patient's or those who are especially close to the patient, makes a clear difference for the kind of talk that goes on. What is this difference?

My conversations with Mr. Oland when he was not with his wife, the patient, were especially revealing of the "difference" in question. Not only was her husband deeply affected by her condition and impending death, but he displayed precisely the sort of vulnerability I have in mind. His distress was an appeal for help—that is, for a clinical dialogue focused on the one hand by that distress and on the other by its source in his love and concern for his wife and his feeling that Dr. Langston wanted to "force things." We reached a point in our final conversation when he conceded that at one time he had been very disturbed at Dr. Langston's words.

> He told me that since she didn't have a living will, and I couldn't tell him anything about what she wanted done, there . . .well, he said he just couldn't or might not be able to do anything for her. Of course, you know, Myra and I had talked some and she did try to get me involved in some of these matters, to get into those things, but even though it was so hard for me to take it or even to listen to her, I still knew what she wanted. It's just that, well, you know, that doctor seemed so impatient with me . . . and all I could think about was how I didn't want Myra to talk about those things, didn't want either of us to think about it. So all I could do is sort of blurt out that I didn't know. And then get all mad, 'cause I knew, though . . . oh, yeah, I knew, and we really agreed; I know, too, she knew that's exactly how I felt, too, but I never wanted her to have to face the thing, and didn't really know that I couldn't take it myself. But there are lots of feelings that are so hard to put into words, especially if you've never had the feeling before, and I just couldn't bring myself to really say what I knew.

"I think I understand, Mr. Oland," I said. "Still, I hope you realize that Dr. Langston really should know about this; he's been very disturbed, too, thinking, I suspect, that he somehow managed to offend you. That's something he'd never want to do. If you want, I'll talk with him, but at some point you really need to talk with him."

"Why? I mean, things are resolved now, aren't they?"

"Obviously, in a sense. But even so, I think it is important for you to tell him what you've told me. He needs to hear it from you; this could help him, and it could also help you, too."

"That's not going to be easy, 'cause things got kinda hot and sticky there for a bit, you know? I mean, like I told Janice, that doctor, I thought, was just trying to force things on us, on me. It's kinda like he was, well, you could say, trying to get me to tell him it's okay to let her go, and I just couldn't do that, not then not ever if I had to do the whatever. I just couldn't live with myself. So, like I said, things got a bit hot, and I even accused him of trying to get me to kill Myra."

"I heard. But, you know, Dr. Langston also felt really bad, even awkward, and he has had difficulty getting things settled in his own mind, too. From what I know he thinks that, but, really, I shouldn't talk for him; he needs to speak for himself. So do you. I can be a go-between only so much."

"I suppose you're right, so I guess I'd best find and talk with him."

Our conversation had then tapered off, and I left thinking about how, apparently, during their earlier, "hot" conversation, Dr. Langston had tried rather aggressively to get Mr. Oland to tell him what his wife's wishes were—whether she would want life supports withdrawn—and grew quite impatient when he wouldn't, or couldn't, talk about that. He just kept "insisting that we 'do everything possible,'" Stan had told me, taking this to mean that Mr. Oland was "confused" and "inappropriate." He was worried that he might be involved in another of those awful cases in which family members push for "doing everything" at a point, however, where "everything" in any reasonable sense has already been "done." Later, he was amazed that Mr. Oland had thought that he was trying to "force" things.[14] In any case, they did talk for some time, and both felt that things had been straightened out.

To my great regret, but as is true in all such situations, I did not get another chance to talk again with any of those in this family—neither Mr. Oland nor Janice, Charlie, or Jennie. I was especially sad not to have talked again with Mr. Oland, who had revealed so much of his grief and guilt and yet so little of his life. Like any clinician, I enter the lives of these people and at some point exit, return to my own affairs, most often without knowing whether my being there made any, little, or no difference to them, there, in their own circumstances. Nor do they know what difference they made to my life. This is the poignant fact of life of clinical work, I know. It is, nevertheless, distressing.

4

Don't Let Me Forget to Remember

Some years ago I attended a conference in Baltimore with a formidable title: "Neurobiological Research with Human Subjects."[1] It was scheduled to last four days. I managed only three. I later heard that, on the fourth day, the organizers hoped that the participants would be able to reach some consensus on some guidelines for protecting human subjects, especially those who are mentally compromised, involved in human research projects. That never happened.

Before I left for the conference, there had been some discussions at my own university concerned with what might be the most productive role that I, as the director of our ethics program, could play in the complex process already in place for reviewing research protocols submitted to our institutional review board (IRB).[2] We were in the process of figuring that out when notice of this conference came across my desk, and, after discussing the idea with the head of our IRB system, we decided that I should attend.

The conference appeared especially intriguing because part of our discussions had touched on the fact that, like similar medical centers, we could likely expect an increase in research proposals focused on neurologically debilitating diseases (Alzheimer's, Parkinson's, schizophrenia, bipolar disorder, and others). Members of our IRB realized that there were at the time no special federal protections for research subjects whose mental abilities are inadequate for them to give informed and voluntary consent or who exhibited variable competence (competent when consent was first obtained but not so at some later point during the experiment—making a later decision by a subject to quit the study at best problematic). I had been asked to help formulate a set of local guidelines, following up on the concern expressed by the National Institutes of Health (NIH) and several major research institutions that research using people diagnosed with schizophrenia, Alzheimer's disease, and other dementias needed and deserved special protections. Just what these should be was, and remains, seriously disputed.

Although Alzheimer's disease was mentioned several times—and, being of a certain age, this was of some interest to me—the conference was mainly concerned with schizophrenia, which on the other hand was of considerably less personal interest. It began to be obvious that most of the participants already knew each other, had in fact confronted each other many times before, and were eager to mix it up in the pitched battle already going on as I wandered in, somewhat late because of airline delays and a taxi ride that didn't add anything peaceful to my frame of mind. The conference attracted not only many researchers, but also a large contingent from patient-advocacy groups around the country who seemed directly and strongly opposed to much if not most of research involving human subjects. This division—researcher versus subject (or family member)—in fact, seemed among the more obvious in the sharp, cutting exchanges.

Several officials from the NIH and the National Institutes of Mental Health (NIMH) were also present and came in for their knocks from both sides—the one convinced that insufficient funding was being provided; the other that neither agency was supporting patient-subjects against the multiple risks inherent in research. Officials from both agencies, on the other hand, apparently believed their role was not so much to answer as to receive the barbs of those who feel the pinch of tight funding or the injustice of flawed protocols and protections for subjects—some of them veteran subjects of such research.

In spite of the announced program, a very different agenda was obviously being addressed: those in favor of research efforts using persons with compromised neurological status against those deeply opposed to this research; those bent on seeking ways to ameliorate the devastation of schizophrenia (and to an extent neurologically debilitating diseases such as Alzheimer's) and those distraught by researchers' invasions of privacy, failures to respect the rigors and requirements of informed consent, or just plain incompetence. All of these perspectives were heard with practically every presentation.

It didn't take very long for me to realize what was actually going on. A bit irritated by it all, my mood contrasted dramatically with those obvious in their disgruntlement or delight at the proceedings, the sundry diatribes and attacks and more. It was rather obvious as the day wore on that some people really thrive on this sort of thing.

I, on the other hand, became increasingly annoyed, sulking even, in my almost silent grousing. *I'm really glad*, I thought, *that I am not one of them*—someone with schizophrenia. The feeling, unwelcome, unwanted, uncomfortable, was perhaps not unlike what John Bradford must have felt as he watched a group of heretics being marched off to the gallows and spoke the memorable words, "There, but for the grace of God, go I."

Nor, the annoying notion began to seep more openly into my awareness, are my wife and children, nor even my close friends, schizophrenic! How lucky am I, how unlucky are they! The thought was neither willed nor particularly pleasant. I recall another part of it vividly: if I were ever to become "like that," I would not want to continue to live; I would want someone to help me die. But not—I quickly assured myself in that sort of silent dialogue I and others may find themselves in the midst of without particularly wanting it to go on—if helping me meant that someone would then get into serious trouble.

But still, there was that thought, that frightening prickle, less vague and more biting the more I let it dwell: even so, would I then want to continue to live? Would there even be "I" then? Not exactly choked by guilt, I admit, it was nonetheless rather an awkward moment, though I had no trouble keeping it to myself.

My discomfort, though, threatened to become obvious to those around me—or so I feared (I caught myself in the midst of hand jerks, eyebrow twitches, enough to make me worried: had anyone seen anything?)—when a psychiatrist (well-known to many there, it was evident, though not to me) who, the one introducing him pointed out, had studied schizophrenia for many years, then began to talk. My musings were abruptly dropped, my attention refocused and brought to the stage where he was wildly gesticulating as he spoke and walked about the stage. His voice was unabashedly passionate and utterly oblivious to the presence of an audience—never mind that it included many research subjects as well as many of his peers.

At one point, he robustly announced without a trace of self-absorption that he himself was schizophrenic and had been hospitalized four times over the past two decades. His experiences as both subject and researcher, like those of several others like him in the audience—though he didn't identify them, it seemed clear that they, too, were well known to the other participants—were a unique resource, he said, that should be recognized and utilized by the research community, including the NIH and NIMH, in particular for service on IRBs to review research protocols on, among other topics, schizophrenia. A remarkable man, an even more remarkable performance! I was completely charmed. Besides, he was absolutely correct.

While I was listening to him, unbidden thoughts and questions nevertheless emerged: What's it like to be schizophrenic, to be like him, much less to be him? Do thoughts "occur" somehow "in" his

mind in the way I think, and say, they do in mine? Are other schizo-
phrenics like him? If I were like him, what would I be or do? Would
I act and talk that way? Would I know what I was doing, as he
seemed to know? Would there be "me" or "I?" Then, remembering
(how or why, I can't recall) that I was scheduled to be on a panel
about Alzheimer's in a couple of weeks, back at my own university,
things really began to percolate, appall, and, a chill running up my
spine, alarm: Could I be schizophrenic and not know it? More likely,
and more chilling, could I have Alzheimer's and *not know it?* How
would I know that and yet not know it? Isn't my awful memory
pretty good evidence? What's it like to have it? Rather, do you "have
it" or "are" you it, or "had" by it? Is there any difference between the
experiences of schizophrenia and Alzheimer's?

It was obvious to me that I really didn't understand much about
either condition, especially when it was put to me inwardly in the
first-person singular. Moreover, beyond the medical, technical
details of Alzheimer's or schizophrenia or other dementias lay the
altogether more grueling and disturbing questions about what, who,
and how I myself would be, if "be" "I" would in any sense, were I to
find myself with either condition. Or, would it be that I "find" myself
or that I would be "found" by others? The questions quickly tumbled
over each other: How could "I" find "myself?" Who finds whom?

Most of the literature I began to gather and read as soon as I
returned home really didn't help much, until I came across a splendid article by Joseph M. Foley, recognized as a leading schizophrenia
researcher. Remarkably, he directly addressed much of the gist of my
by now somewhat frantic musings: "What do demented people experience? What does their condition mean to them? What is their
reaction to it? What are their gratifications? What are their frustra-
tions? Does dementia allow the development of coping strategies
available to other people with afflictions?"[3]

I was brought up short, for here was a key example of those creeping, creepy notions that had oozed up into me from some primal
existential mud, dreadful and alarming, during that conference in
Baltimore.

Think about that awesome, altogether appalling condition,
"dementia," or simply the word, "demented." What *is* it like to be
demented? Does a person with schizophrenia or Alzheimer's or
Parkinson's know that he or she is demented? If so, how does, how
can, a person deal with it? If someone is "losing it," we cutely say,

does this then mean that he or she is no longer able "to deal with it?" Do they even know what they are now or what they were before?

And for that matter, how about people who, for whatever reasons, take care of demented individuals: who *are* they now to those who once loved them, sharing inexpressible intimacies? How must they now feel and think and act? How do they get through each day? Would I, or you, want to live with, or be obliged to take care of, someone who is demented?

Dr. Foley bluntly squares off with just such questions, for they are, he emphasizes, among the most commonly asked and the most urgent. But, they have yet to receive any "satisfactory answers"—and he asks, "Why not?" Indeed.

Years ago Janet Adkins, a fifty-four-year-old woman in Oregon, was diagnosed in the early stages of Alzheimer's. At the time, she was among neither the elderly nor the infirm. As most of us learned only much later, after what was apparently considerable discussion with her sons and her husband, Mrs. Adkins concluded that she was already at the point when she was just beginning to sense, inwardly I suppose, that Alzheimer's was beginning to have its insidious way with her. She and her family decided that she should go to Michigan to see Dr. Jack Kevorkian, the retired pathologist whose name they had first heard during a meeting of their local chapter of the Hemlock Society—the famous, or infamous, "Dr. Death." It later became widely known that she had become the first of Dr. Kevorkian's steadily growing number of cases of assisted suicide.

Janet Adkins: hale and hearty at the time she made that fateful decision, but with what she and her family believed was a bleak and brittle future approaching ever more closely and rapidly, with nothing to stay its stubborn course. She sought out what seemed the only alternative—if "alternative" is even how to talk about this—to retain some control over her life in the face of Alzheimer's sure, gradual, but always menacing onset, the overt coming about of what seems, all things considered, the most dreadful of anything. Which was not death so much, of which we can know nothing anyway, nor yet only dying, so long as the pain can be curbed or tamed, as Mrs. Adkins is reported to have insisted. What, then, is so dreadful?

I hadn't read Dr. Foley until some time after the conference and hadn't put any of it together with Janet Adkins or Dr. Kevorkian. All I had to go on at the time were those insistently wormy thoughts and gloomy feelings.

I realize, of course, that I'm not alone in having had such an experience; others, many others, apparently also find such thoughts slyly quickening unbidden in the bottom of their souls or minds, especially on occasions when someone with schizophrenia or Alzheimer's, or someone caring for "one of them," appears and in their very appearance insists on being so oddly compelling. And, all along, this ghastly whisper inside me: *I'm so profoundly glad*—smug and snug might be the truer thing to admit—*I am not demented, am not going through that dreadful, detestable experience.* It was at that point, and closely tied to it, that the other notions came creeping in an ever so ominous way into my awareness.

The one was about John Bradford—that "there, but for the grace of God, go I" business. But the other, too: what *is* it like, what does it *feel* like, to undergo dementia, to go through being demented? And what is it like to find yourself in the early stages of one of these debilitating diseases, like Mrs. Adkins, when you know something's out of kilter or is going to be irretrievably askew, then later when you don't know anything? When there seems to be no longer any "me" to know or say anything, no "me" to recognize itself or anything else?

And, unavoidably, the other horrific thought: how can you take care of, care for, a person who doesn't even recognize you're who you are: wife, husband, close friend, son, daughter?

All those musings, that story with its dreaded theme of becoming demented, are mere preface to a second, briefer, all but equally unspeakable tale.

I went to have a checkup on a Monday afternoon not long after I had returned from that conference. A Doppler ultrasound had been recommended by my personal physician because he was not "comfortable" with what he heard when checking out my right arm and my right carotid artery running like life itself up that side of my neck—straight up, of course, to my brain, that seat of my "what I am."

He wanted to check out the right arm because neither he nor his nurse were able to get a good "read" on my blood pressure or pulse on the right; only my left arm yielded the wanted messages. He said, "You need to have that checked by Doppler ultrasound. Let's see what's going on up there."

Okay, let's see, I thought, or actually, I took it rather passively, without much thinking I realized a bit later on. But, reflecting back on that experience, I was already beginning to sense a creepy shard of ice moving up from somewhere in my stomach. My own schedule coordinated with the Doppler folks, and we were on—"Just to check," he said. "To make sure all is well."

At about the time I learned when the Doppler tech would do her thing on my neck, I began to get a bit nervous: "bad news," I had it all figured out, meant that I would be at serious risk of a stroke, and one likely result of a stroke could be losing a good bit of my, what? Self? Mind? Soul? Spirit? Brain? Alertness? Anyway, "I" could be in difficult straits. Because of all this and, doubtless, that Baltimore conference, still very much with me, a bristling bush of notions stridently mounted up from the basement of my psyche, my self, my soul, my whatever: of a sudden, there they were, those appalling prospects, demanding, clamoring for attention. I could lose my mind! No, not that, but the more appalling, my mind could be lost and, with it, myself!

I was still alright, though, I thought, for I still managed to hold it all back; small and fleeting, my shudder was barely noticeable, the short walk, unaided and unwavering, to the place where the deed would be done, the awesome message recorded and reported; then I could—I *would*, I swore to myself—go on about my life.

Calm, then, I was, but not for long. First, I had to go down, down to the basement of the building. (Why are these machines always in some wayward, veiled place out of sight of the usual walk of life, down, too, where few people mill about?) And with each step down, that imagery of basement—cellar, vault, crypt, subterranean forces in the service of the nefarious and ill willed and the like—grew ever more menacing and I more chilled.

To add to it all, before I went down to the vascular lab for the Doppler, I mistakenly went to the cardiology clinic, where I presented my clinic card (precious as gold, you know; even more so nowadays when managing and competing for our very personal health as commodity has become the name of the new medical insurer's game) only to be informed that I was in the wrong place and would have to go still further in the basement of the clinic building, around still more deserted, isolated, corridors, or so it seemed as I walked, inched my way apprehensively to the correct locale, with all those haunting, eerie feelings and thoughts newly erupting, unasked for but seeping up nonetheless, as I stepped up to the counter: "Doppler Ultrasound Sign In Here!" the sign was flagrant in its naked display.

There was the vascular lab. I introduced myself, said what I was there for, and, digging about for my clinic card suddenly realized that *I didn't have it!* If no card, no Doppler, no needed news; that's okay; but where the dickens did it get to? My pockets yielded nothing, but I kept clawing my way through first one then another.

Obviously, it occurred to me, the woman at the cardiology desk hadn't given it back to me—except, I had this clear recollection that she had indeed given it back. So where was it? I rummaged through all the available pockets in my wallet, pants, shirt, jacket—as anyone would do in such circumstances, I assured myself.

Nothing.

Now—the other side of the insidious is the utterly open, I kidded myself—I won't have to know, for I won't get the Doppler, since I don't have the card, and I don't care where the damned thing is! And, that's just fine with me! Not knowing seemed just fine!

But, that's not what I said to the woman at the vascular lab. I said rather that I couldn't find my card, I had just had it, gave it the person at the wrong desk, cardiology, and now couldn't find it, and now what?

Hopeful, eager, anxious. But, she just said "not to worry," and promptly dialed the cardiology desk, found out that my card had been returned to me before I left that desk. So where was it? Not here, nor there: surely the woman upstairs was mistaken; she had obviously misremembered. The picture is easy to conjure. No mystery there. We've all had such inconsequential, petty lapses, right?

Then, suddenly I had one of those sickening, spine-tingling icy shards of feeling explode: if I got the card back from the clerk, put it away, then it should be *somewhere*. I mean, every card has to be somewhere, right? But I can't find it: and the wily, treacherous sense stood there, like something right out of Poe's wicked imagination: *Am I slipping?* Is this perchance an early sign of that dreadful, dreaded fading-away of me, of what I am?—*Alzheimer's?*

I don't know if any of you have ever gone through that sort of experience; I know it happens to me more than I really, truly need or want. Once is quite enough, you know. I've never had much of memory anyway, so people tell me. Now, however, such lapses seem not only a bit *too* frequent, but also invariably carry with them the grisly hint, a faint whiff, of dementia.

Incidentally, I never found the card; the folks at the lab kindly had another made, totally destroying my growing hope, wish, urgency to get out of that place, rest easy once again in the blissful terrain of not knowing such things as I might learn there.

Truth is, I don't want *that* to happen to me! I don't want that to happen to anyone in my family, either! I don't want. . . . Why not?

What is it like to be demented? De-mentia: losing it, your *mens* somehow slipping away; what happens when that happens? What disappears and where does it go? Maybe *wits* is the better way to say it: wits, which suggests humor and at the same time covers the ballpark of the mental and the soulish: acuity, perceptiveness, intelligence, but also desire, volition, emotion. I, and I think each and every one of you, would really like to know, to understand, to have some insight into: what is it like when you lose all that, those wits? You no longer *mens*, mind, as you are now de-mented, de-witted, de-minded. Can I lose my soul as I apparently can lose my mind?

But also: how can people with Alzheimer's, schizophrenia, or any other de-mentia be helped? Who can or should help? What do or would you do to help?

That sort of questioning abruptly brought me, anyway, up against an oddity with unambiguous bona fides: I, who now (presumably) somehow possess or otherwise have *mens*, I can "mens" with the best of them, I am "minded" or "witted;" I have my "wits" about me, we say; or I haven't yet lost my "mind."

Now I find myself wanting; I need to understand what it's like to become de-minded. Does that make any sense: I who have my *wits* intact want to know what and how I would be if I were to lose my *wits?* Psychologically, what do we experience when we experience the utterly unknown, what can't be known since we, would-be knowers, now no longer have the wherewithal to know? Is this what it's like to ponder something almighty: I, simple, mortal, finite, imperfect, how is it that the very notion of the infinitely, eternally complex, the higher and the perfect, can even enter my *mens?* Wouldn't the utterly unknown, supposing there are no word games here, be then impossible to experience? And can I, or you, think even, without some experience of some sort, no matter which? Like death, perhaps, never itself experienced? Hence it is that thinking and knowing, like dying, really are so puzzlingly problematic.

At the time, I wasn't sure just where that link of ideas would have taken me; nor, frankly, am I now at all sure. I do recall several lines, paths, doors invitingly opened up. And, confident now that my memory is still intact, still gives no evidence of the onset of anything de-menting in myself, I find myself wanting to go into one of those doors, to test it even if only a little.

First, the very idea of undergoing Alzheimer's or Parkinson's, of becoming "de-minded," seems all the more chilling and foreboding in view of their characteristic, ever-so-gradual onset—of whose ominous course each of us would surely be aware, however much we might want to wish it away, understandably. That knowing-ahead-of-time, ahead of *my* time, unlike so many occasions when it may seem great to know something ahead of time, is in this instance just the reverse: deeply appalling, a time for panic.

The idea of losing my mind—more to the point, I now think, losing my what I *am*—is as terrifying as it is awesome. For what is ultimately threatened is my very own sense of my very own self, not only my "what" but my "who." This is a threat that, Eric Cassell once wisely observed, is surely key to what suffering is all about[4] and just as surely reveals a good bit of what Janet Adkins must have gone through and be a close part of what eventually took her to Dr. Kevorkian's ramshackle VW bus with its makeshift manner of "assisting" her dying, ending her still-undemented life and mind and soul. Not to mention countless others wasting away in dismal nursing facilities, or the back rooms of houses, abandoned, all of them, by the ones whom they care about most and now know, intimately, that they are not themselves cared about any longer by them. As my mother once said, before going into one of those forlorn places herself, and even more fervently once there: this is a prison, plain and simple; and to make matters worse, they treat you like a child.

This brings to mind reflections by Robert Terry, a physician specializing in caring for those with Alzheimer's, who some years ago was moved to write about the disease. He came to think that the real affliction of this disease is that it *removes* you from yourself. He says that it strips away "your very humanity, your intellect, your personality, your personal habits of hygiene." However lethal other diseases may be, by contrast, they do not "turn you into a vegetable"—as Alzheimer's and other dementias invariably do if the afflicted individual lasts long enough for the dementia to lay full siege.

Dr. Terry's message is clear: there are indeed things worse than death, for becoming demented is far worse than either death or dying. Possibly worse than extreme pain, it may be. Sure, we will all die at some point, "but," he continues, meditating now in the first-person singular, "I don't want to be destroyed as a human." To become demented is to lose precisely what defines me as *me*, this person I am: me-myself-and-I, we learned to say when we were still children. But then Terry goes on: Alzheimer's "lessens our humanity," and because of this, he thinks it is at least understandable that "mental disease is—was [regarded as] sinful. That's because it changes our very soul, our very spirit."[5]

But just here, reading these words, I had one of those inner hesitations we undergo when something seems just not quite right. Wait a moment, I thought, is it that my *humanity* is muted, lessened and eventually lost, or that *I myself*, my *soul* or *spirit* is muted, lessened, and then faded away—and then what? Does it move, go, to some *other*, nether place? But in either case, *where?* And, with barbs aplenty now, *how?*

In some ways, at least something of what Terry alleges seems in a way unquestionable: some diseases do strip away cognitive abilities, alertness, awareness, even the capacity to relate with other people. In this respect, it may be said that they cancel, vacate one's very self and personhood. But do they also "lessen our humanity?" If ever "I" am no longer "me," does this mean "I" am no longer "human?"

That is troubling: does the loss of a person's faculties signify that his or her "humanity"—and thereby, it must seem obvious, what gives us a moral status, if not the moral order itself—is *therefore also* lost? So that, it would then have to be supposed, while it may be wrongheaded to think that mental disease is "sinful," to lose "our very soul, our very spirit" *is* to be effectively wrenched outside the moral order. At least as an active moral agent. For, to be within the moral order is often thought at the very least to signify that one can and does choose, has reasons for those choices and is capable of taking responsibility for those choices and their aftermaths. To the extent that the capacity and exercise of rational choice, at least in some part, defines our humanity, then to lose that ability must therefore place the individual beyond the pale of moral action, agency, and accountability. Is all that correct? Does this story about my own inwardness, my self, my world, get it alright?

In effect: does losing your "soul" or "spirit" mean the loss of your "humanity?" Or is it the other way around: losing your "humanity" signifies the loss of your "soul" or "spirit?" But does losing either or both also mean the loss of moral status? Is what makes an individual a moral agent (choice, reasoning, acting, assuming responsibility) equivalent to having moral status? Saying "yes" to that seems a bit harsh; maybe, even, there is a sense in which there's something fishy, fallacious, even ominous in such words, implications that were probably never intended by him.

Which brought me to a second line of thought. Several things come to mind in trying to sort out what lies beneath Dr. Terry's otherwise discerning observations. Isn't it after all evidently true that something quite profound, perhaps definitive and even constitutive of what each of us *is*, is indeed somehow lost, or somehow becomes no longer present, no longer effective, is no longer recognizably *there* where that person *is*—when a disease like Alzheimer's lays full siege? And if that is so, then aren't my queries and ruminations little more than nit-picking?

Or is it otherwise? Consider: what Terry expresses seems evoked for most if not all of us regarding those who've become de-mented. Yet, if that be so, then don't our typical responses to people with Alzheimer's really come down to the idea that, however deserving of pity, and their families of sympathy, those who are demented—because "they" are no longer with us, but have lost it all—therefore just *don't matter*, they no longer make a difference for us, they are no longer of "our world?"

Truth be told, for most people today the de-mented just don't count as much as the rest of us, whatever the cause and etiology, as the ways in which we typically "manage" them, in institutions or hospitals or at home, demonstrate. In our charge, we shunt them away, we who have been fortunate enough not to have our wits stripped away by injury or disease and have somehow managed to keep our wits (or so we like to think and anxiously demonstrate to others).

Not that there is no reason for this behavior of ours, because it is rather less peculiar than it may seem. After all, the question can't be ignored: how is it possible actually to take care of and to care for a person once close and loved who is no longer "there" and who no longer recognizes who you are and who, often as not, cannot seem to follow through on even the simplest of orders?

What at some point becomes obviously different about them—when the demented, whether because of Alzheimer's or schizophrenia or psychosis or retardation, become a literal *them*—is enough different to make a difference. Most often, they're no longer part of what counts as "the moral community." Why? Well, isn't it because they are or seem no longer able to conduct rational discourse and interactions as you and I understand these, are no longer self-determining, are thus seen as no longer responsible even for their actions? What else would anyone need?

But, apparently, to follow through with these ruminations, to affirm all of that is to wind up endorsing an ethics based mostly, if not solely, on the notion that persons and only persons are true moral agents and as such make up the moral community. And is it these rational agents whose job it is, in part, to turn right around and define what counts as "moral" and therefore who gets included and has moral standing in that community? As David Smith observed,

"At some point someone entering into a dementia begins to count less than, or have a different status than, the rest of us." Not only that, for he goes on to propose that "personhood hinges on the ability to accept responsibility. When that ability has disappeared—when it no longer makes sense to blame someone who is careless, inattentive, or out of touch—then there is no longer a person, and we should speak of a diminished form of moral, and perhaps legal, status. . . . [I]f you cannot be praised or blamed, you can't make quite the same moral claim on us that people we hold responsible can make."[6] So, it would seem, I must be in error, my understanding flawed regarding Terry's words, for not only does Alzheimer's strip away your "humanity," it seems to Smith, it also in the same way filches your place in the moral community.

Does this make sense? Do the demented count less than the rest of us, the nondemented? Or, is that widespread, deep-lying sense of no longer counting, no longer needing to be reckoned with, expressive instead of a deep malaise within contemporary society: we do think less of them, *but should we?*

Here, only utter candor will suffice. In my own musings about schizophrenia, Alzheimer's, and the like, I, too, found myself with a feeling that seemed to underlie a murky but disturbing thought: that were I to come down with that abominable disease (or be grouped among any other of the "de-mented" and "de-witted"), I would become to myself somehow vile, less than I was, less than what made me "human," no longer the "person" and "self" I was and, if no longer, then desperately needing to be again, impossible though that be—an impossibility that in turn feeds on the passionate denial of being "of that sort."

And, suddenly, a third line of thought began to appear: are "person," "self," and "human" the same? I once went to great lengths to demonstrate a significant difference between "self" and "consciousness." Is that same care needed here? Is it really true that to be afflicted with Alzheimer's is to become *less* than human? If you or I now became demented, in whichever form, is it in any serious moral sense somehow to be then *less* deserving? My brother, say, now with Alzheimer's, is he *therefore* no longer, somehow, the same as once he was, at least in that he is no longer "human" and no longer within the moral community he once was, before he came down with that dreaded disease? However demented he may now be and however dim the prospects of his ever recovering his wits: is he not indubitably, unquestionably still deserving of my care, respect, love, concern, help, whatever is needed and whatever it is that "moral agents" (even as "rational persons") as such deserve? Even more, indeed, for he is my brother—for now how long is it? All my life! He is still, is he not, that same brother I once had, though now he is himself (he "be's himself," if I may, as in the old expression, "I be damned!") very differently, and who, for all his older-brother attitude to me, the younger and therefore never equal, yet always nursed and nurtured me when too often it was I who got cut, scraped, broken, and always managed to hurt myself. Is he not still that same brother who laid low any of his own friends who would put me down?

Having that shared history, my brother and I, commits each of us morally to one another. Is not the very relationship itself a moral phenomenon, with moral standing? And, if only one of us remains who can still understand and commit, then aren't I, when he's demented, all the more responsible to understand and commit? Or is it otherwise, now that he is—if he is—no longer "human?"

Is human dignity really tied to nothing but the full, rational, moral agency many people today think is the very base of ethics: autonomy? If my brother, my father, my uncle—any of them now in the grip of a dementia—can no longer be "self-determining," is any of them thereby reduced, now less than fully moral, as Smith apparently says, backed by Dr. Terry and so many others nowadays (for all that I find of real value in their writings)? If a person is not, or is no longer, or is only variably, autonomous, then *is* he or she any longer within the moral order? And, even if perhaps still included therein as deserving somehow of moral concern, is he or she then to be treated as no different from, say, a lively monkey or sturdy sheep?

I wonder how I now would conduct myself with my brother if he now no longer recognizes me.

And if I think—as Smith, Terry, and others would have me think, with all the good intentions with which I wish to credit them—and if I still love and have fond memories of my brother, what does that way of thinking say about him, my brother?

One's ethics may say far more about oneself than it might say about what's right or wrong, good or evil. At least, I should think, the source of my brother's moral importance must lie in him, not in some status the rest of us would confer on him. The problem may lie with us, in our too-eager focus on "autonomy" and too-little emphasis on him, on them, on those others who are undergoing that appalling loss of a sense of self and the ability to know the others who yet not only love them still, but know how much care they both need and command.

All that seems so robust and confident, which it doubtless is not, but it led me then, and now, to still further reflections. Dr. Foley emphasizes how utterly individual it is to be demented. While some patients "are aware . . . that they are in intellectual decline" (an awareness that can in some individuals persist even into later stages of Alzheimer's), he says, others become openly hostile to any suggestion of the least mental slippage, and some are utterly unaware that anything at all is happening to them. Between the poles, Foley remarks, "are infinite variations."[7] Like everything else human—ethics, politics, religion—Alzheimer's is ineradicably unique and individual. In Foley's measured words, "Each patient, if we are able to delve deep enough and long enough, will have an individuality that will elude any of our efforts to find the 'typical'."[8] And, it might well be appended: if we but have patience enough to be with such patients.

So rather than worrying about the "moral status" of fetuses, infants, comatose, or the demented, apparently, Foley wants us to learn to be focused on other matters. First, what and who are we, anyone who dares to ask "what is it to be demented?" What do my actions, thoughts, and feelings say about me, and is whatever I say and think and do, is this the sort of thing I, or any of us, really want to leave as my, or our, legacy?

Second, if I would understand and care for a demented person, there's nothing for it but to plunge ahead to encounter fully each unique individual, in his or her own unique circumstances, with all the differences from myself and my situation it portends.

What does any of this say about ethics? Well, in a way, that's both easy and very difficult to get a hold of. In Foley's words, "If we are going to talk about ethics in relation to dementia, we must know not just about cognitive capacity but also about awareness, feelings, and emotional reactions to the personal and social consequences of dementia."[9] But then, only a bit of modest deliberation is needed to recognize that you're always with individuals.

Which goes straight to the heart of it, so far as I can see: it makes us appreciate that the really basic ethical questions are, no matter who you are and whether you are demented or not, *who am I?* And, with that, *who are you?* Which means that "ethics" is a matter not so much of "moral status"—which, all things considered, seems to be only too open to the possibility of a political power game, only in appearance unlike what Thrasymachus claimed—but to the contrary, of multiple and complex relationships between and among individuals, you and me and him and her, but also they and those over there, and still others, who find ourselves asking, or being asked, the awful, awesome questions of who we are and ought to be singly and together as we grow older, making whatever music we can with one another.

And ethics—is it not?—is invariably a matter of having to probe into and within each individual situation and circumstance, for each of us is, Ortega y Gasset wisely reminded us, one who can say "myself-and-my-circumstance," even while each of us displays that remarkable and ungetaroundable ability to be inside oneself.[10] May this not be what is suppressed in dementia, this ability to be inside myself? Diverted, as demented, instead to the outside, to what approaches whether in danger or not, we are forever alert to any and everything *there* except ourselves *here*, and that is maddening, if not madness of some order.

We need, in ethics, to probe somehow into each individual life and, with Ortega, those circumstances, in order to learn what and who is or was that person, now demented perchance, but utterly human and, as David Smith, despite what he has already stated, does say, is utterly deserving of all our loving, caring attention.

It is that *regardless* that is commanding. It is that *regardless* of which I must always be mindful. Dignity is not the same as moral agency, but rather, in Smith's more fitting words, "dignity is foundational, and human dignity is distinctive, but its root is our engagement with one another, engagements that are often most deep when the issue is nurture or love."

As came to me in the course of undergoing the experiences I related earlier, *relationships* are the centerpiece for ethics. Smith concludes, "Although we should not treat [demented persons] as if they were not demented, we also should not pretend that they are no longer part of our family or community"[11]—which goes in quite a different direction than what he averred about moral agency and moral status. Which is fine, for gets it closer to the truth, so far as I can see, for it keys in another significant, if largely unstudied notion: to treat people without pretense and *regardless* means that *respect* is the strict correlate of "dignity," not, as often assumed, of "autonomy."

For those of us fortunate enough not to have become demented—dare I say "yet?"—some of us will nevertheless have to live with persons with dementia. Likely, in light of the fact that the population is aging more and more (me along with the rest!) we will all have at some point to live with someone senile or demented: to face and live with those who will at some point no longer recognize us, regardless of how intimate we once were, yet who must now somehow be cared for.

And, this, like the other reflections, also returns me to myself, to who I am or ought to be for and with all the others in my life: "As the need for care is universal," Richard Martin and Stephen Post urge, "so the provision of that care is a part of the fabric of civilization. Caring for the dependent young, the infirm, and the aged is essential humanity, a biological reality tantamount to breath."[12]

I am left then with the powerful, even ominous, sense that I might unwittingly cease to care for the least and most suffering among us. And if I would become that person, I would do so on pains of ceasing to be civilized and thus ceasing to be a moral being. And this, I remind myself, far more than being demented, would cut me away. In a word, again, I am called to respect, to live that *regardless.*

There are people both expert and sensitive who have undergone the experience of caring for people with dementia, and their reports are both heartening and disheartening; their courage admirable, the responsiveness of the community too often far less. Yet, I find myself inwardly hesitating, and unwittingly (the point intended at this stage of my musings) reminded of my latest foible with memory lapse. If ever I do come down with a dementia, hear me now: pay attention to *me*, whether I am aware of what's going on or not; don't forget *me*. Somewhere in that terrain most intimate—as regards whatever it is whereby I am aware of myself and am myself with all my "parts," my infelicities and untoward attitudes—there is also the most haunting and terrifying: not death, not even dying, but that who I am will no longer be, *nor will I know it* while yet the rest of all this I call "me" will remain to be fed, housed, clothed, washed . . . *by whom?* And I, more deeply than I had ever thought possible before, do not want that, not that for my wife, my children, my friends, not even for strangers who might nurse me. That, the thought comes to me, would just be too much, too much to ask or expect any of them to have to undergo, even as I recognize that I would, I think now, not hesitate to do that for one I love. Can I let another do that for me? Is receiving as morally significant as giving?

The figure of Janet Adkins returns ineluctably to haunt me, even entice me: why not, if ever the first signs of madness begin to occur, get rid of myself? But hear Mrs. Adkins: it was not for her sake (pain, abandonment threatening to flag her resolve to be brave, and such), but for the sake of her husband, children, friends. She simply could not put them through all that. Her motives resonate with me, for I don't want my wife, son, daughter, or close friends to have to go through having to care for me.

But, the piercing question erupts again, this time to bitter presence here: is it truly within my power, my ability, my wish to "get rid of myself?" *I* can do *that?* I know the moment I think the thought that Kierkegaard is right there, grinning just around the corner over there, knowing this special form of despair is itself the subtlest, most intractable source of despair—not so much, or only, trying to rid me of myself, but what it must mean to rid me of the . . .

Perhaps it's true, in Smith's words, that "as humans our lot is to suffer together."[13] But, for all his sincerity and loving kindness—and he does have that and more—I wonder if I will ever find in myself, there where such things brew and boil up, such thoughts that are more than thoughts? It comes to me in this moment that I in my deepest self know that there may well be something "worse than death": that, having to do all those things for me when I lose my wits completely, or even for some time, what my family and friends would then have to do for me. At least, having such thoughts and feelings as these be conjured up in me, I begin to understand, I think a little better than before, just what and why there are Janet Adkinses nowadays, and, yes, even a Jack Kevorkian here and there.

It may be our human lot to suffer together; as long as I can do anything about it, I shall in any case try to help others in their suffering, and to suffer with them and, hopefully, they with me. I have—as I'm sure others have as well—such a hard time bringing myself to be the one for and because of whom such suffering by others must occur—and this, I begin to think, may be a powerful argument, if such is ever needed, for the centrality of love, of care, of concern, in ethics. With that, I want to move away from Janet Adkins and others who found they had to have that fatal visit with Dr. Kevorkian.

And then, I come to still another pause: Who am I to say, on the one hand, that I, we, must still care for those who are become demented, for they have not lost their place in the moral order; who am I to say that, fatefully, on the other hand, not I—oh, no!—don't care for me that way. Is this not the epitome of selfishness? So, must I now go on to recognize that I, too, must, if gripped by whatever dementia, be prepared to receive and accept (even, with desperate secrecy to want) the care of others? That I must learn now to *receive* and not just give? Has our "ethics" been too riveted on giving and too little on receiving?

I find myself in this curious, odd dialogue with myself quite a lot these days, as I age. And as it goes on, something otherwise dormant begins to surface. I said I had experienced this sense—embarrassing, inept, all that—that I was "lucky" not to be schizophrenic, so far as I know neither demented (and the other thought, unavoidably: would I know this?) nor yet on the way to it (would I know this, either?).

"Lucky?" How odd to find it expressed that way in me (I cannot claim to have thought it that way, only that that's the way it came up in me). Or it may be not so strange at all. Survivors of serious accidents go through something like it, I'm told: even though felt as deeply immoral, even revolting, yet they report the thought, "I'm glad it wasn't me!" Which turns John Bradford around: "There, thanks to the grace of God, goes he, not I!"

And yet, that's not quite what's now running through and rising up. No, something else. That, rather than my own "good luck," true though that surely is—my life marked with far more "good luck" than "bad"—there is an even stronger sense of utter outrage that *anyone* would have that utter "bad luck" of dementia. How could that happen, what is this accident—all the more intolerable because it seems mired in the multiple accidents that is anyone's birth—this outrageous assault on a person with a slow, gradual loss of that very sort of self I sense in me and know in thee? Or, if not accident and there is a God, then how could we possibly dwell within an understanding that such things are, despite God, yet here and to be lived with somehow? If, the classic expression of it would say, God is omnibenevolent and omnipotent, then the merest, the slightest suggestion or whiff of evil (Augustine's lamentation over having stolen a pear when he was a mere child) becomes ontologically the deepest and most problematic of anything, not to say theologically paradoxical.

And that thought, powerful and decisive, whatever else it does for me, evokes an equally decisive and powerful response: that dementia, unasked for and undeserved, is cosmically *unjust*. It ought not be. But it is, and since it is, so must I respond by doing all I can to undo its caustic marks, to undo what has now befallen you, my comrade and fellow being:[14] I must help you, ease your pain, assuage your suffering, ensure you are never abandoned. And, with that, I know, is the other half of that thought, that recognition: I must prepare myself to be not merely giving, but to be on the receiving end of those giving care, if it be me, not thee, who falls to dementia.

5

Broader's Hill[1]

"No question," Dan Knox muttered to himself, "the car has got to be put in the garage soon, but that means getting in and driving it there, and that means someone else has to do it, because, the thing is, this game is just now getting interesting, the guys just might get it on this time."

Which is just the sort of thing you might have heard if you'd been around that afternoon when he was lounging in his favorite chair, the TV humming, and watching the ritual Saturday late afternoon NCAA March Madness basketball game, him thinking about then rejecting the notion that his brand-new car really should be washed. It was really dirty, dirty still from the jaunt he and Alex, his just barely teenaged son, had taken the evening before, after Alex got out of school. They just had to take it out on those dirt roads, test that great suspension and awesome tires. But Dan just didn't want to get up, so he told Alex to get the Trans Am and bring it up the long driveway to the garage, knowing of course that nothing could keep Alex from a rare chance to get behind that wheel all by himself. Now, Dan mused, if only he could figure out how to get the same reaction on chopping those logs outside into usable pieces for the fireplace.

Alex was on the shy side of fourteen, as was his good friend, Jase, Jason actually, who lived next door, best friends forever it seemed, and who just happened to be standing out there by the car just looking at it—jealous? admiring? Icy delight shivered up Alex's spine.

Jase saying, sure, hell yeah, man, he'd like to go for a short ride in that bad Trans Am, all red and even just sitting there seemed already winged like a fighter plane he once saw at the air force base. Maybe, the thought occurred at the same time to both of them, we could just mosey on down the road and get a coke and burger at the DQ. Alex's dad only recently bought the car, his wife Betty still wondering why since, after all, the old one, not even old really, still got from point A to point B.

They got in the car and, sitting wide eyed, Alex put in the key and just backed up and out of the driveway, but really that wide-track red car purred off to what was supposed to be only a brief spin to the

DQ, on country roads all the way, where no cops would normally be found, them both underage and all. The narrow two-lane ribboned asphalt wound around the sharp hills and abrupt valleys for three or four miles around their houses, before emptying right where the DQ was, then connecting to one of the several major arteries to the city some forty miles away.

They came up over the first of several turns up on Broader's Hill, the road cutting a brief, blunt turn up again then a short sheer drop down into a valley. Alex felt the car suddenly lurch somehow out of control. He tried to cut the wheel hard to the right, to compensate, but the car felt instead like it had a mind of its own, and then—oh, oh, God, what's happening? The car veered precipitously left, spurting and twisting off the road, then back the other way, then a jolt and nothing.

Probably, if you'd been able to witness the thing, Alex lost control, maybe the car's tires ran over a boulder, hit a pothole maybe, or something while he was paying anyway too much attention to Jase, talking, goofing, thinking about hanging out and looking cool at the DQ, and instead the new red supercharged Trans Am, roaring tires spinning off the pavement, pitched, wobbled oddly on one side, then flipped the other way, how many times is not clear, maybe only once, while the slow hot afternoon sun freeze-framed each grinding crunch of the car, each collapse of fender, and each flailed arm of whichever boy, sun glinting off that roof and a jagged piece of glass.

Alex was flung out of the suddenly open door, his loose seatbelt never hooked, and landed mostly unhurt, in mud the way it sounded, but knocked out, too, as the car still tumbled, coming to rest in a ditch with maybe an inch of water slowly flowing down the hill to the west. Several small trees were pulverized, the car itself not as mangled as you'd expect.

If you'd been there you'd have seen the open moon-roof with one small body sticking out crazily, arms akimbo, head cocked at an odd angle, feet not visible, still caught inside. You'd have seen how Alex sort of parachuted into soft ground, but Jason, a raggedy doll, was pitched violently. You might have wondered how that slight head could withstand at all that jerk and crack as the car, dense enormity, stopped almost on top of him and left you wondering how or whether in all that ghastly crunch of metal and tree and solid earth Jason could yet still be alive.

Not even Alex knows if that's the way the accident actually happened, even though he was driving. He's not remembering much, and nothing at all about the accident itself. So, we're all left to wonder and guess. But we know, too, there is no remembering for Jason.

What we do know is that a young man, age about fourteen, was admitted to our hospital in mid-February, due to what was described as a "rollover MVA"—a motor vehicle accident where the car rolled over at least once and probably more than that. The ambulance crew arrived on the scene without knowing how long Jason had been unconscious nor how long he had not been breathing. The note they left at the hospital said, in part:

> 2/14: 14 y/o male involved in rollover MVA approx ½–¾ hr ± (?) prior to EMS arrival time, circa 6:45 P.M.; presumed partially ejected from car sunroof with body half still in car, feet caught in steering wheel, pat. found supine, pupils dilated and fixed, no pulses, motor response, on arrival; neg. pulses, neg. motor response, pupils fixed, agonal respirations on EMS arrival, intubated, IVs per EMS. Multiple contusions w/abrasions. PEA—bradycardia.

When I first became involved in the case, I remember wondering, as I usually do, what had happened, what had brought these two young men to that place and time when and where the accident happened. You almost never know someone before they appear in this or that unit, with this or that illness or injury; nor do you know much about what they were like before, much less what happens after they leave. So, I almost invariably find myself wondering about the patients and families I meet and, when I don't know much, I usually find myself imaging what it was that brought them here at just this time in their lives.

So it was with this young man, Jason. I had heard that another young man, the same age, had been driving, which means too young to be driving, trouble on wheels. How did they get in that car? Had they stolen it for a joyride? Were they drinking? Using drugs? What? A bit later, before I began to write all this down, I heard something about the case—probably only hearsay, because baseless rumors circulate all the time in hospital corridors—that the kids had been in the father's car, the father of the one doing the driving, the one who was not especially hurt, giving the situation more than a little touch of painful irony. And, hearing that, my imagination took over, playing out several different scenarios, each of which took them to that place on Broader's Hill, where the EMS crew reported the accident took place and, I mused to myself, the last place Jason would ever have seen.

Also, when I was first asked to consult, I looked into the medical chart and learned more about the situation, at least what had immediately preceded Jason's admission to the trauma unit. I kept my own notes. By that time, for instance, he had been hospitalized for almost a month before I saw him and read these notes:

> Intake trauma nursing note: 2/26 P.M.: Pt ejected from r/o MVA and crushed by vehicle w/few to 0 life-signs, resuscitated and intubated at scene, tr'd to med center by copter; driver also, but preliminary checks out ok. 2/27 A.M. Post intubation, intravenous fluids, and restored blood pressure at scene, pt tr by helicopter to med center. NG tube + ET tube in place; C-collar on neck; lungs clear to auscultation bilaterally.

> ER physician note: 2/27 A.M.: Sedated and comatose no motor movement noted; large degloving laceration right occipital region; pupils 2 mm non reactive & equal; right eyelid ecchymosis; right ear laceration through lobe to cartilage.

So, here was a young man who had been severely brain damaged in a rollover car accident, but otherwise surprisingly undamaged. I heard indirectly about the police report that the driver had been thrown clear and was relatively unhurt, while the boy in the passenger seat— well, this was Jason. Clearly, his brain was just about ripped off his spinal column, as one neurologist's note all but stated:

> Neurologist note: 3/1 A.M.: CT scan of head: some blood along tract, some pneumocephalus; severe scalp laceration seen superoposteriorly; right posterior subgaleal hematoma . . . gray-white matter differentiation poor . . . sulci somewhat effaced bilaterally . . . subtle areas of diminished density within frontal white matter . . . ventricular system somewhat small . . . right globe proptotic, right intraorbital contents otherwise unremarkable . . . evidence of cerebral edema . . . subtle ischemic or non-hemorrhagic shear injuries.

As I glanced through the chart, several notes stood out. For instance, just prior to being discharged to the pediatric intensive care unit (PICU), the emergency physician wrote:

> ER physician note: 3/1 P.M: Plan: continuous cardio-respiratory and neurological monitoring, intubations w/ vent support, sedation, CT head, chest, abdomen, ICP monitor placement, labs as indicated.

Then, soon after Jason was transferred to the PICU, a nurse wrote:

> PICU nursing note: 3/4 A.M.: Past medical history noncontributory; allergies: no known drug or other allergies—EEG flat, no cough, gag, response to deep pain suggest that if pt survives

it will be in veg state only. Temp 100.4, respiration 20, BP 136 to 159/73 to 88; non reactive; jaw wired shut, abrasions noted and treated.

Not long after, the attending PICU physician on duty at the time had met with the family, with the consulting neurologist, and several nursing staff there as well. The former wrote:

> PICU attending's note: 3/9 A.M.: Family conference w/attending and chief neurologist to explain results of scans and deterioration of neuro systems; told them pt may progress to brain death or end up persistent vegetative state.

There was, however, nothing said about what the family thought, said, or felt. Then, a bit later, one of the PICU nurses recorded Jason's medical condition just before the consulting neurologist came by with his team to check him out:

> PICU nursing note: 3/16 P.M.: No reported hx drug use or abuse, no alcohol use or abuse, no indication of use or abuse by test or clinical exam.

> Neuro note: 3/16 P.M.: CT exam: cerebral edema noted, may resolve . . . possible focal left frontoparietal cortical hemorrhagic contusions, but difficult to differentiate from artifact . . . worsening bilateral maxillary, bilateral sphenoid and anterior left ethmoid sinus disease. Would recommend DNR status and discussion of possible life-support removal. Prognosis dismal.

The social worker then assigned to the PICU (and, as in so many hospitals, other units as well) was regularly seeing both the family and the patient. As it turned out, there was more than one "family" involved, as the parents had been divorced and both had remarried. From what she found, there was little or no animosity between the two new families. Indeed, both Jason and his older brother (by one year), Jack, had spent a good amount of time with their father, who lived a considerable distance away. The social worker wrote at one point:

> Social worker note: 3/21: Pt's parents reported divorced x8 yrs; pt and older brother have lived with father and step-mother, but recently moved in with mother and stepfather. Latter family wants to help take care of pt (tracheal cleaning, changing diapers), and father's family would like to do so as well if needed. Might consider tr to rehab facility.

If such a transfer could actually be arranged, and if it made medical sense to do that, the social worker told me right after I became involved, then none of the "problems" that prompted the consultation request to me in the first place would be present; they would instead be the rehab hospital's responsibility then, she said. I found this shifting of "problems" quite disconcerting, said so, but knew she was in any case correct: there would be a transfer if this were medically feasible, whatever I thought or didn't think. Still, I resolved to put in a call to the rehab hospital, if only to alert them and let them know I'd be willing to visit if they wished.

The consult request came shortly after transfer had been raised as a possibility, so I didn't have the chance to raise objections or questions; it was a done deal, and all I could do is ask about it when I did finally get involved—which was on the twenty-second of that month, the same day the very involved resident had just recorded the results of her exam and raised the idea of an ethics consult:

> Resident's note: 3/22: Pt comatose, no oculocephalic, corneal grimace, flaccid quadriplegia without response to noxious stimulus, pupils non reactive, positive corneal bilaterally, positive doll's eyes which are improved, no facial droop. Spontaneous breaths began 3/20, no spontaneous movements; assessment was severe hypoxic injury. Suggest ethics consult to ensure family understands implications.

The attending then wrote, agreeing with the resident:

> PICU attending note: 3/22: Overall prognosis dire and DNR status discussed with family. Given pt's lack of cough and gag reflexes to maintain airway patency and lack of ability to turn or ambulate, DNR seems appropriate but family upset and refuse, want aggressive pulmonary toilet, and prompt response to any cardiac event continued. Ethics consult requested to discuss issues with family.

But, beyond having the nurse manager place the call to me, the situation had not changed much. Except: the day after I was called and had my first talk with the mother and the boy's step-father, both agreed that a DNR—do-not-resuscitate—order was appropriate.

But not a word about a DNR order, not even whether the attending had discussed the matter with the family—as I had asked in my note to this attending. This was not some sort of major faux pas; it happens all the time, and from all I can tell for reasons that are credible enough to take some of the air out of any complaints I might have voiced. In this instance, the attending told me when I asked her about it that the mother, "though she certainly gives every indication of understanding what I told her," was "just not ready." I understood, I think. It takes time, sometimes a lot of time, for people, parents especially, to accept this kind of news. But things were not getting any better. I talked with the consulting neurologist that day, and he confirmed in no uncertain terms his sense that continued treatments of any sort, including the feeding tube, were "inappropriate," and he insisted that a DNR was "needed, absolutely," stating that there was "no way" this patient could be resuscitated, given his neurological condition. In fact, he had written a note, and repeated it to me, that the "prognosis remains dismal." No quibbling there.

And, several days after this, the attending did write the DNR order:

> Ped. attending note: 4/2: Physician's Order to Limit Cardiopulmonary Resuscitation.
> This form must be completed in full, including legible signature.
> Code Status:
> DO NOT RESUSCITATE—In the event of cardiac or respiratory arrest, all cardiopulmonary resuscitative efforts should be withheld.

> Attending note: 4/2: DNR noted and signed by parents.

> Resident note: 4/2: DNR in place, talked with parents, they seem to understand.

Several days later, the medical chart continued to record the dreadful news:

> Neuro service note: 4/8: Profound coma persists and no signs of recovery; gag and cough remain negative; no spontaneous movements; MRI demonstrates (1) increased T2 signal throughout basal ganglia and (2) contusions in frontal and parietal cortices. Progressive encephalopathy from hypoxic-ischemic encephalopathy and shear hemorrhages. Recommend discontinuation all supports. Pt does not yet meet brain death criteria but appears to be deteriorating in that direction; prognosis remains grim.

The family continued to have serious difficulties accepting this prognosis, however, and the resident who had been with the case almost from the beginning noted their refusal to discuss discontinuation:

> Resident note: 4/9 A.M.: NB pt's relatives, esp Mom and brother, still excited when pt closes hands (reflex grasp), opens eyes, etc. Explained that does not mean alertness or awareness, only

involuntary, reflex movements, and that eyes-open coma the worst kind for prognosis. Still not sure they grasp meaning. Call neurology for another consult?

Then, recording what would eventually keep things from going on and on, the attending noted what nursing staff had been suspecting for some time: Jason's lungs were just not working right, and were in fact beginning to freeze up, causing respiratory problems that could not be resolved:

> Attending note: 4/14: Pt is 13 y/o s/p, r/o mva 3/14, PEA, and anoxic brain injury; no spont mvmt, no resp pain, no cough, no gag, no posturing. DNR status cont'd to date, acute episodes hyperventilation ➞ severe atelectasis continuing/progressive, prognosis grim.

And the inevitable occurred within two days. The day after that note was written, the resident had rotated to another service. Because of her considerably greater experience with Jason's condition than the new one, however, she was asked to come back "asap" on the sixteenth. She did, and wrote:

> Resident's note: 4/16 , 8:20 P.M.—no longer on that service but called emergently to bedside by nurse who knew me from before. Pat. suffered acute episode of hyperventilation + dusky color observed by nurse and RT; bagged by RT but hyperventilation continued assoc with resp distress.

Then, a few minutes later, it was over. The resident noted that death was pronounced at 8:53 P.M. and that the patient had died of respiratory arrest. Though the cause of the arrest was still a bit uncertain, the resident suspected atelectasis and probable embolism. This was later confirmed. Her final note read, in part:

> Resident's final note: 4/16, 9:00 P.M.: Pat. became acutely apneic & by time I got to bedside pat had no peripheral pulses, and HR 35 by auscultation. Over next few minutes, nurse said she thought pat had expired; I returned to bedside and confirmed no HR, no respirations on auscultation x1 min.

> Attending final note: 4/16: I have reviewed and confirm Dr. Parton's note and confirm the patient's death. Family is currently at the bedside; discussions about donation may be initiated again, if they desire; check re autopsy. [Signed] Susan E. Rochelle, M.D.

It was the nurse manager (in my notes known merely as "NM"—the medical and nursing practice of writing, and sometimes even speaking, in acronyms was infectious; or, it may be, I was just getting some revenge for being labeled the local "CE"—clinical ethicist), who first called me about the case. While I had been actively engaged in such consultations for almost twenty years, I had slowed down somewhat and had instead been immersing myself in the world of biomedical research. The change was so that I could try to understand this world, and I felt I had to immerse myself in it just as I once plunged into the foreign climes of clinical encounters so as to understand the what, which, how and why of concrete moral issues in clinical settings. I was thus clinically involved only when covering for one or both of my colleagues—which happened at the time of this accident, when both were vacationing at some distance elsewhere, thus unavailable. So, Helen, our administrative assistant at the time in the center, sent the call through to me, thoroughly disrupting what had been planned as a quiet day of writing.

Here's what I jotted down after the nurse's call for "someone in ethics."

3/24: Asked to see family of Jason Knight, a 14 y/o boy involved in a single-car MVA some weeks prior with a friend who was driving and was reported ejected from the car, which rolled and wound up pinning him underneath for an unknown time. He was unconscious at the scene, never regained consciousness, and is currently (circa six weeks since adm) PVS [permanent vegetative state] or close to it (according to what the consulting neurologist on case told the Mom and wrote in chart; "PVS" not actually used, nurse manager [NM] says; Mom told Jason is "dying" and won't make it).

NM notes plan to transfer pat. to rehab facility is on agenda, and caused Mom and current husband (name?) to ask neurologist why? Why put him in rehab if he is dying? Neuro response gives me problems: to cover all doubts, in essence. To make sure Jason is given every "chance." Which isn't exactly what he otherwise told the parents—something about the "ischemic injury appearing as if yanked out of its roots, like the stem of a mushroom, frayed but still attached to its top." Plus, NM's emphasis, neuro also notes "hypoxia" from prolonged absence of oxygen.

Agreed to meet Mom and Dad-in-law next morning. After some confusion (see below), I held the meeting, included Mom and her sister (pat's aunt, from Montana); Dad-in-law joined a bit later. Mom uncommonly alert, considerably intelligent, and uncharacteristically realistic; clearly a caring person, but devastated and in much grief. Mom and father divorced for 8 yrs (he lives in Portland, OR, but has flown out several times already, and plans to repeat visit as often as needed). They have joint custody, and she emphasizes how well they all get along; in fact, Jason lived with his father for some years before coming to live with Mom and brother about three years prior; more, there are frequent phone calls between kids and Dad. NM says Mom having difficulty accepting idea of DNR and that Mom initiated call for a talk with me. NM informed attending and resident of my expected involvement.

I went to the floor (NB: pat. now out of ICU and on regular peds floor) to meet with Mom, but she wasn't there (turns out she was down at cafeteria getting coffee). Consternation: discovered I didn't know her name, found chart at nurses' desk, learned it is Janet Knight. Looking over the chart to familiarize myself, especially with what neuro had written, discovered that a DNR *had* been written (with the red notice on the page and on the cover). This made me call NM, who told me that at 5 P.M. Mom had agreed, and had talked with her former husband, boy's father, who agreed as well. Looking over the DNR, noted that the first box had been checked (no cardio-pulmonary resuscitation).

At about 10, Mom came in and I met with her and her sister; later, Mom's husband arrived. In considerable grief, yet unexpectedly articulate and alert to what is going on with their son (and aunt's nephew). Able to focus discussion very sharply on current and anticipated decisions to be faced. First, the DNR was not exactly what she understood: she does not want Jason intubated and connected to a vent (now he's only on nasal canula with moderate O_2 reading, but basically breathing on his own). Second, unclear whether transfer to rehab will ever be done (possibly tr to home instead?) and if it is, whether the DNR will be honored—that is Mom's question and needs answer. Also advised them to be similarly clear in advance of any subsequent transfer. Mom concerned that Jason not be brought home (answered the question before I had a chance to ask it); says she couldn't handle that, especially with Jason's 15 y/o brother also at home (this for further discussion). Third, after much discussion of "dismal prospects" (they deliberately cited neuro) and likely outcome (PVS, so it seems, again cited neuro), they were advised to be thinking about what to do: hospitalization would likely not be required after a few weeks, and Jason had to be tr'd to some other place.

They were all surprisingly reflective and well informed; Mom even brought up Cruzan situation, which I took as implicit permission to discuss very candidly nature of questions and decisions likely to be faced in future: d/c life supports (expected request for a trache, anti-biotics, suctioning, feed tube). They asked whether they had the authority to withhold all treatments from their son, even asked about feeding tube, though Mom clearly anxious about that; she mentioned other son "very angry" at her when he learned she had signed permission for DNR—I agreed to talk with him if possible (he may not want to come in). I promised to talk our own attorneys about d/c supports, esp. feed tube, but advised them to learn as much as they could from an attorney of their own choosing. Fourth, although the father said to be in agreement with DNR (even saw total withdrawal as looming—must discuss these matters with him soonest), I noted that this had not been documented—I promised to contact attending and neuro on this matter as well.

In the face of profound tragedy, Mom and her husband are remarkably alert and tuned into issues, able to discuss very difficult, awkward matters without losing sense of their son and his plight. Highly unusual. Both expressed gratitude for chance to talk with me, promised to page me if needed, and I promised to get them the clarifications needed.

3/25, I got neuro by phone and he agreed (1) to discuss the DNR with Mom in detail, and (2) to call father and document his oral agreement (per my concern that Mom be alerted to the possible unhappy future of his disagreeing and accusing, etc.). Actually, however, I detected no animosity whatsoever between/among of the principal parties; nothing but good things said by each of absent others; hence, common sources of conflict, subtle or not, seem not present; keep alert to these, however, as this situation harbors potential for explosive issues.

3/26, I called and talked with hospital attorney by phone. I asked the awful question re PVA and minor child and parental decision making: do parents have the legal right to make the decision to have feeding tube d/c'd? Told it is not clear here re withdrawal/withholding of life supports in cases of pediatric terminal condition, nor about removal of feeds in such cases. His advice: have a conference with docs and parents if/when that eventuates; and, please, include him! Asked him to contact NM and inform of interpretation and worries.

3/26: Called NM to let her know what I had been doing and learning. She told me Jason not tr'd to rehab, at least not yet (mucus plugs still occurring, plus still has need for higher O_2 than rehab will accept, etc.). NM will discuss w/Mom, re the business of need to discharge from hospital soon; Mom now thinking, on advice of social worker, about tr to some other facility; maybe even eventually to home (she can surely be readily trained to manage, all believe). I'm on call.

I tried any number of times to figure out just what happened and why. I knew by now that there was no stolen car, no drinking, no drugs. Did the father's car have a tire blowout? Did Alex, inattentive as kids can sometimes be, not see a pothole, or a boulder, and, hitting it, have the steering wheel jerked from his hands? Or did he yank the steering wheel, perhaps showing off, and lost control? Without drinking or drugs, what made the car crash and roll over? Granted, the kid shouldn't have been driving anyway, but kids do that, and parents often let them do it. And disaster is all too frequently the very next thing that happens. Moreover, there was the fact that both Alex and his father—mother, too, no doubt—were really shattered by the accident, and I wondered all along whether there was anything I could say to either of them. Was it Alex's fault?

I could not let this one go. Maybe it was because the boy's mother and father, though divorced, were so obviously bright, and wretched, after the accident. Maybe it was because it had not been very long before all this happened that my own son had been in high school, just beginning to drive and all, when he, too, had an accident. Not very serious, it turned out, but I knew then and know now how chancy such things always are, how it could so easily have happened very differently from the way it did. I knew how our lives were willy-nilly lived out in the midst of chance and how we are forever making bargains with this or that deity—"If you'd just, . . . then I'll . . ."—or how we beat and berate ourselves—"If I had only waited just ten seconds, even five, then . . . it wouldn't have happened!"

Jason could just have well have been my son, I knew that and know it now, and maybe that's why I just can't let this one go. Stuff of nightmares, I know, and I do wish I could stop it, or even just mute it all.

So, I found (and still find) myself playing that "what if" game many of us take up. I knew, for instance, what Alex was going through, and the anguish of his family, but "What if," I have often mused, "Alex had not really been at fault? What if he couldn't help what happened?" Could he and his family get through any better? And, not knowing, none of us, precisely what happened out there on Broader's Hill—I've since driven out there more than once, but silence is all I hear—then shouldn't I maybe play that game out loud, so to speak, tell them, Alex too, that it wasn't really his fault? No one knows what actually happened, and I came to know too well just how awful Alex and his family felt, so would I have been wrong to have made something up, all the while just trying to help?

I didn't. I told them instead only what I knew, which was not very much; we then just discussed what I had heard, some of it from them in fact, that the police reported that the car had gone out of control, that Alex had lost control and . . . well, we're human, right? We all make mistakes, or bad things happen to good folks all the time, and, well, that's the way the ball bounces, the cookie crumbles. How can we live and make sense of our lives in the face of the awful happening of chance events?

Even today, though, I can almost actually hear the squeal of those tires as Alex jerks the wheel that's gone out of control, then the crunch of metal against solid ground in the cool of that evening out there on Broader's Hill, then the creak and slight snap of the cooling engine. I can almost feel the sizzle of hot metal, smell the reek of leaking gasoline and the stink of smoking tires and exhaust, at this moon-chilled and oddly vivid scene.

It's almost as if I were actually there, witness to the horror and quite as unable to do anything to stop it as I would have been had I actually been there.

Later, when I had done what I could in those discussions and conferences, much later I thought I heard another kind of call go out, for help, too, in its way, because Jason's mom and dad and others in this family, like Alex and his family to be sure, were all caught in unmitigated grief. This became so clear when they realized, made real for themselves, that Jason just would not "make it," would actually, really and truly die right before their eyes.

And none of us, myself included, had any of the favorite words at hand from the common tongue, but were instead baffled, too, by the idea of Jason's death. When it actually happened, his final breaths, when that resident came rushing down from her other unit to be there, to be with them and with Jason, it all became awfully true, so true they hurt to the depths and wouldn't stop. No words could in any way ameliorate. This boy, Jason, even if he was just out on a joy ride with his buddy, Alex, is now so close to death there's nothing the doctors and nurses can do to save him, to bring him back, his brain all curdled in a final closed and taut ball of incomprehension, unfeeling, unawareness, final coma.

His parents know for sure now, as certain as can ever be, that Jason is certain to die, to go through the final spasms of breathing, clutching hand, with that doll-like look that is no look at all, just flattened out there on the bed, and there's nothing either parent can do to stop it.

Asked about donating Jason's organs, neither of Jason's parents, Charlie and Janet Knight, know what to make of that, can't quite hear it, can't see mind's-eye-like to know what's being asked of them, nor is either able to focus on any of that, although they had—like others—talked about it, it must have been ages ago, and even applauded that story on TV that night back in January about the family that'd done that, donated not just one but all of their dead child's organs. And how much better they said they felt even if still in the grip of anguish and grief and loss, how that act, that simple "yes" could make you feel as if some part of Jason would live on, in some other's body who might otherwise have died, and that's a good thing, isn't it? Still, neither of them could shift to that, neither could more than vaguely associate even the noises with words, it seemed a foreign tongue or no language at all.

Nor could the doctor, Dr. Susan Rochelle, help much, gentle and kind woman though she clearly was. She was, of course, very experienced, though entirely new to the medical center and hospital, having spent her career to date in private practice. Moreover, she was very uncomfortable with everything; even though no spring chicken, she simply had no experience with this sort of issue—DNR, removal of life supports—none at all with this sort of thing. Maybe, she said to herself more than once since coming on to her monthly rotation on the service, it was a mistake to come here, maybe she should have stayed in that town she had grown used to and had actually begun to like, never mind what she had also told herself and made her contact her old friend here in the first place. It couldn't get much worse than what this poor family now faced, the Knight's grieving so deeply, wrenching her heart; but she just didn't know quite what to do, in the most practical way. She'd never withdrawn a ventilator—hardly ever, in fact, had a patient on a vent anyway. "Damned cars," she said to me one day while we were having coffee, "bad as smoking for teens anyway," vowing to keep her bicycle.

"How in the world can that person from the donor agency talk about donating Jason's organs, just tell me that," she went on, "I

don't know how they do it, I know I couldn't do it; if I had the accident, I'd never donate my organs, though I should, I know; studies
show it works, but somehow it all seems so ghoulish. And how about
you? You do the same sort of thing, don't you?"

She wasn't asking me for an answer, for she went right on: "Yet
there they are, the Knight's, apparently agreeing to the idea of
removing the feed tube, and I've got to stop this somehow, don't I? I
mean, you can't just take that away, can they, can we, can I? I know
they want it over and done with. If they can't have Jason back whole
and entire, I know they want it over, and so do I, so do we all, for
God's sake, but we've gone way beyond the point where that's even a
small point of light. But can a feeding tube be withdrawn?"

"Yes, that's clearly the thing to do sometimes."

"From a kid, a minor?"

"You know, Dr. Rochelle, you might want to talk about these things
with Dr. Arpress, you know who I mean, the pediatric oncologist?"

"I've heard of him, but we haven't met yet."

"Well, it might be a good thing to discuss these issues with
another physician, one who has had lots of experience dealing with
situations like this one."

"Maybe so, maybe so." Her eyes grew distant, as if focused on
something neither I nor anyone else could see.

Which I took as a good moment for me to excuse myself and leave
her with her thoughts and fears and feelings. I went back to my office
and called Dr. Arpress, whom I knew fairly well, to let him know that
he might be hearing from Dr. Rochelle and what it was about.

"The problem," indeed. Just what was it? It wasn't just a matter of
removing the ventilator. That wasn't what was bothering Dr.
Rochelle. Rather, it was the haunting question, whether a feeding
tube could be withdrawn from a child, a minor. For the real "problem," in the end, was just that: not only the awesome difficulty of
removing a feeding tube from anyone, but removing it from a
child—and not just the fact that Jason was still very much a child, but
the actual, practical act itself: How to do that?

As she had said, "If he were just still on the vent, we could disconnect that and that would be that? And we could even ease things so
that there wouldn't be too much agonal breathing. But a feed tube?
I'm sorry, but that's different. Isn't it?"

I begged off, although I knew the answer—clearly, it is permissible
to do just that if a minor patient is ever in Jason's sort of condition—
I also understood that "difference" Dr. Rochelle emphasized. What I
told her instead was that I'd check with the hospital attorney right

away and let her know, so that at least the legal issues would be clarified. I did and reported back to her: all our attorney insisted on was that it be very clear that the parents agreed and that he be there when it was actually done.

"I'll try to tell the straight of it," Dr. Rochelle told me after I mentioned the attorney's sense of things, "but also can we give them some space, some tiny bit of room for hope?"

"But is there any room for hope?"

"No, I suppose not. It's just so damned tough, but I'm still going to give them some more time, somewhere between a few days and . . . and what? A week? How long will it take, I just don't know and they expect me to know, and I have to tell them my best judgment."

"They can't expect more, I should think," I said, but she hardly heard a word.

"Can they understand any of this without being doctors, too, and knowing that we, I, just don't know how long? I know that's okay, that's the way it is sometimes, just so long as you're not asked to speed things along. But I've got to put in some drugs, some pretty lethal stuff when you think about it, to help that poor kid with agonal breathing, and keep the parents and family out of the room, out of the way altogether, they shouldn't have to see what I think's going to happen, it won't be pretty. Anyway, I know I've got to do it, I just want to keep them from seeing the awful part of it. So, can you help with that?"

"Of course, I'll do whatever I can, and I'll talk it over with them, too. Maybe I can find out if they have any questions, any they haven't had the wits to ask yet."

"So, okay, then, it's settled, or almost. I'll give it a couple of days, and you talk with them, that's fine, that should help. And thanks, too, for putting up with me now."

And when the time came, everyone—mother, stepfather, brother, one aunt (mother's sister), father and stepmother—awed and hushed in the face of what was needed yet seemed so impossible.

A nurse edged over to one of the nurses from neuro, whispering furiously, "He's almost brain dead for God's sake, right?"

And her reply, I could hear, "Not quite, and isn't that the whole problem?"

"My God we can't kill him, you know?"

"Shush," someone says. "The family is right outside the room now."

Someone else's words coughed up as if from some hypogeal source, a voice but whose I couldn't tell, said "Even so, we all know that there are times and people willing to act, to do what we all know is the right thing, right?"

"The right thing, right, thing, right?"

And someone else, never knowing for sure anytime just who said what, pointed out that the chart was "odd." Odd how? I wondered, and was answered: "Well, even with the DNR and DNI, and all the talk from Dad and Mom, you know that there's no note about the tube or antibiotics or anything else? You know?"

"Do we have any choice?"

But just as someone went off to find Dr. Rochelle, I heard the nurse back in the room abruptly let out a sort of sob. And I knew, just knew, that everything was over, had to be, people don't make that sort of noise otherwise, and I then knew or felt I should have stayed on, if nothing else, to witness, for a witness was surely needed at just this time, with that long and agonizing process, that impossibly drawn-out dying over all those weeks in that terrible bed. Jason's death seemed drawn out way beyond expectations, beyond even the expectations of physicians more experienced than Dr. Rochelle or the resident whom the nurse had called in to help at the last moment.

Jason somehow managed to die, his lungs doing little more than making a bit of room for some blood clot plunging through his body's final arteries, plunging through until, in the tiny space the lungs nudged open, the clot came on and that space closed and—pulmonary embolism, they say—it stuck, lodged in that narrow place and his lungs could no longer do what was needed. The family meantime grieving so deeply out in the hall, waiting, stupefied and gripped by the horror of it all. Then they came into the room and held onto Jason as, finally, mercifully, that embolism, blood stuck, artery plugged, did what had been so desperately needed but that no one could be found to do.

I stayed on through all this, awed by it all, Jason especially, I stayed there in that room to witness as perhaps none other could or would, watching as that pitifully small body lurched a bit, his chest sunk in on itself, while the monitor made its sharply drawn up-and-down zigzags on the screen, convincing testament that life still lingered there, but only lingered. Until finally, imperceptibly almost, the up-down scrolling blip bounced first a little less, then with an almost audibly mournful sound it stopped, it flat-lined, flat and only a line, no up-bumps or down-drawn signs of any life at all, now none, no more, none, no signs, finally definitively dead, now.

As I said, I don't know how this young boy got himself in that fix; how the car, driven by Alex, turned over and over, winding up on top of Jason. I don't know how long it took for the ambulance to arrive at the scene, nor who called it. I don't know where the boys were first taken. I don't know by whom they were seen at the accident site, nor what was said.

I do know, but only indirectly—through Mom, stepdad, aunt, brother, medical chart, several physicians and, later, the boy's father—something about Jason before the accident: "He loved soccer." "He was great at math." "His new girlfriend, Sally, is really pretty." And, after the accident: "He was hard to get a bp on." "He looked okay outside, less than what you'd expect, but you knew he'd really hurt himself bad." And the clincher, "The main part of his brain seems yanked out of its roots, like the stem of a mushroom, frayed but still attached to its top."

I also came to know something about the family, Jason's daily condition, and other matters more directly, as I talked with family members and their close friends, physicians, nurses, the nurse manager, social worker, chaplain, and others. Becoming involved in situations like these is invariably coming across countless allusions to countless "elsewheres": other ongoing events, people, and relationships (past and present, but also hoped for) that ineluctably insinuate just how much is going on I neither know about nor can reckon with in the course of listening, talking, and the rest of it. These hint at and hide details and issues in sometimes perplexing or bristling ways. These shade and set off conversations with everyone involved.

Talking with Mom, however straightforwardly it may be, is haunted by indirections and inklings of other times, wisps and whiffs of places and people, clues and tracings faintly suggesting hopes or fears, ghosts of people not there but so obviously important for this family, for Jason before the accident—whom I'll never meet, yet who were, who may have been, significant for all their lives: for how they feel and think about ethics and God and politics and farms and the weather and movies and school and doctors and hospitals, how they came to believe whatever it is they believe and with whatever passion it may be, secrets never revealed and apprehensions they may have that can't be spoken aloud. Does it matter that Jason, loving math, was also failing English? That he was caught attempting to steal at a jewelry store earlier this year? That he lost his virginity earlier that same year? That he dreamed of becoming a musician? That he had begun to play a trumpet? That he harbored ill thoughts of his dad?

I had a brief conversation with Dr. Rochelle about Jason's first arrival at the ER and heard the merest suggestive whispers, inaudible almost, of kids and cars and girls and beer and too much teenage sex, and why the hell can't the damned politicians do something about this or that. She talked to me in her soft way, but I heard, as if beneath and behind and between her words, far harsher things almost clamoring to be said out loud. Yet there it is, acrimonious accusations biting between the sounds of her words, crinkling her lips, narrowing her otherwise pretty eyes—more bleak, even harsh, belying her quiet words. And I think of what must have been going through her mind, behind those eyes, in that silent way we have when listening, even intently listening, as others talk and we follow the panoply of emotions play on and around and become displayed by face, hands, arms, legs, torso, head tunings, noddings, fingers doing an impatient dance.

Watching Jason's head loll about on the bed as a nurse cleans his arms and legs, I am troubled and find myself thinking of so many of those subtle insinuations of who he was, slight intimations of what he might say about his likes and dislikes, his fears and hopes, what he might feel about being in this condition, how he talked with Alex in that car and what they said to each other, whether Jason said something just as the car crested Broader's Hill or Alex's attention wandered at just the wrong moment.

Joe Burnowski, Jason's attending in the PICU, was a gentle and obviously caring young man, often described by nurses as bearish in his frequent hugs, not long out of his residency. He is clearly deeply troubled by Jason, his condition, his dad and mom, by what they say to him. And my first hints of, how to say it? Vigilance? So many of the key players in this awful scene seem so vigilant, on the lookout, but for what? They seem like sentinels, but why? Alert and tensioned, yes, but what for? Is it that Jason's brother—Jack, he's called—flying in the face of all the evidence, is somehow heedful of Jason himself, not that shell merely but the boy himself? Can Jack somehow hear what others of us cannot? Does he know something we cannot know?

Mom, too, contrary to everything she's been told, seems expectant, mindful, but I'm never sure of what. It seems almost as if she's desperate for the merest of signs, any gesture, that will announce a significance: "Hey, Mom, I'm really here! I can't talk but watch my hand . . ."? Mom is watchful, brother, too. But so are nurses and—the thing that prodded me on this path—Joe Burnowski seems tense every time we talk. He's on a bit of an edge even, gentle and courteous and kindly though he truly is. Wary, maybe guarded, as if he, too, expected Jason to wake up at any moment. Is this what feeds mom's vigilance, too? Have others in the situation picked up on this central figure's jumpy and almost bodily watchfulness as somehow significant of potential recovery? Is this body language I'm witness to, and is it so potent?

Am I dreaming, fantasizing, merely guessing, puzzled as I am by this? That mom—she especially—is so bright, intelligent, articulate, plainly knowledgeable of what's going on medically, neurologically, yet is so captivated by those neurological tics and twitches on her son's face, his hands' faint neural spasms, fingers seemingly clutched, so that she just can't bring herself to acknowledge what her intelligence on the other hand tells her is the only reasonable conclusion? "Mom can't yet accept . . ." and "she's in denial." Lord, how often I've heard that, and wonder every time what it can possibly mean. Of course, mom doesn't want it to be true, that Jason is on the edge of death. Of course, she looks for the tiniest of the tiny signs. Who wouldn't?

I wonder not why we don't or can't say what we mean to say, but in whatever we say, what else is also said. People perfidious even in the midst of seriousness, of utmost purpose. Language treacherous, speech disingenuous, words deceptive as ice: never meaning what they say, never saying what has to be said, yet hoping against hope that someone, anyone, can hear it said.

Look at how we treat—too often just plain fail to treat—people in serious pain, chronic pain all the more. It's uncomfortably noted in the most professional places, even lamented, how difficult it is to get a grip on pain, to study it scientifically, and why? Why, because it is so damnably *subjective*, so profoundly me and mine: what hurts for one is a mere blip for another, who may nonetheless feel the most hurt when its locus is not the leg but even the slightest twinges in the heart.

But if you really hurt, is saying so then a lie? So obscure that it can't be understood? "On a scale of 1 to 10, how much pain do you feel?" But why a "scale," all neatly numbered and . . . false? And, not knowing how to get a grip on such subjective feelings, such wily and wildly variable feelings, we wind up hardly ever treating pain very well. People, too, sometimes.

So, is it alertness to possible pain, to Jason maybe hurting still, even with his massively damaged nervous system; is it that to which Dr. Joe seems so vigilant? Does he maybe suspect something else than life there? Is he busy interpreting furtive, abstruse signs of things not quite seen or seeable by others but that he, despite that, experiences, apprehends, in a way even understands, and is expectantly awaiting, knowing all along what they suggest, what they are leading to, as these otherwise recondite signs inevitably hint at other not-yet-seeable events: death it may be at the end of it all. Jason dead, no longer there but merely body-husk, cadaver? Dr. Joe, watchful, observant, yet circumspect too, especially when he's around any family members. Yet, as I watch him watching Jason and see him seeing mom, don't I see too something peculiar? He's truly on guard for something, that cautious touching of Jason's head, neck, chest, alertly listening with his stethoscope to . . . what? To something that infused and maybe infuses that life, waning yet not yet altogether absent? Is Jason dead? Nothing left of his presence here save for that still oddly trembling finger?

Is that what the nurse also senses? I can only guess, so clever is she in not revealing anything by lips, eyes, cheeks, not even head nods that would otherwise let us know what she might think of it all. Yet as she manipulates Jason's arms and legs, reattaches bags of nutrition to, drip by drip, feed this body, almost husk already, with its daily dose, is she also sensing his not quite being completely gone but being far enough into death for her to say, "Hey, it's time to quit all this?" Do the good doctor's gestures and cautious words not really display the horror of what's just about happened already, even while those words belie, if you're really listening, his guarded talk? Has Dr. Joe ever been in such a situation before? Are there other vigils lurking behind his vigilance?

Doesn't Jason—for all the ischemic and hypoxic injury to that most fabulous of organs, his brain, therefore his wits, his . . . what? His soul? Spirit? The meat of who he is or was? Doesn't Jason, anyway, still reside with us, if not in that almost cadaver on the bed, then somehow nonetheless an occupant in our hopes and fears, in our very vigilance? Are these mom's thoughts as she caresses his forehead?

Then, unbidden, I think while watching her of Faulkner's *As I Lay Dying*: if Jason *was* Jason, *is* Jason not still Jason? Somehow? How does *is* become *was*? Watching Dr. Joe and Mom softly murmur, I hear Faulkner's Darl, Dewey Dell, and Cash—oh lord, yes, Cash—as he tries to empty himself for sleep, but cannot, cannot "empty himself for sleep because he is not what he is and he is what he is not. . . . And since sleep is is-not and rain and wind are *was*, it is not . . . yet, I am *is*." Is? *Is* Jason still there? And if he is not, is he *is-not*, like Cash says it? Is this *is* only, then, *was*? That's what Jason *is*. His "is."

"My *brother* Jase? How *could* you, Mom?" I hear Jack even now, or so I imagine it had to have been, there, in that hall next to Jason's and his bedroom, in that house. "How could you go along with his death?

Didn't that kill him? I touched his *hand* and he gripped *my* finger, Mom, grabbed me almost like he used to! Don't you love him"— and, soft and brittle beneath all that, "Don't you love me?"

I can just hear him still, now, in this moment moaning in his sleep: is this what will happen to me too? We are all tiny children in the face of the massiveness of this accident, this tiniest of moments when alertness faded, and that car careening, crunching. Is this what this family willy-nilly faces now, each day, from now on?

By the time I was able to look at Jason's medical chart, I felt already that daunting sense of moral pathos: how little will I ever know about Jason and his family, the doctors and nurses, the EMS people who first rescued him—is *that* what they did, "rescue" Jason? How little, yet how immense and imposing are the words that must be used to grab onto the questions they must answer and the issues they must decide, they cannot help but decide.

And for me, too, how pitifully little will be what I will come to know about them, yet how momentous the decisions I am there to help them reach, reach out for, knowing how slight the grounds for making those shattering choices. For Jason, of course: his destiny already decided by what happened, sure, but that will never assuage or belie their grief or guilt, nor my sense of failure, of plain inability to help at all. But also for each of them, this family, doctors and nurses as well, each in their own unique ways and within their own singular lives. Vast oceans our words conceal: "outcome," "result," "aftermath," "decision," "choice," whose soul heavings will not ever, really, never be finished, over and done with; not really. Even though the sheer passing of time will in fact fade sharp edges, heal much, and well. The "once only, once, and no more" (Rilke running through my mind) that it happened, here, with this boy, in that car, on that hill, at that time, bathed in that eerie light; here and now, that once-for-all-time happening will yet happen forever, will go on endlessly happening.

As, too, doubtless, will my own meanderings in these fields, these ineluctably perilous places where we have our once-and-only lives.

And Jason? Where is he now? Is he *only* was, even as he echoes through my constant memory? Where was he when I watched, vigilantly (I admit it!), his mom caress his forehead, his brother put his finger into Jason's palm, the nurse alert to any signs of anything. Jason? What is he now?

6

The Cruel Clarity of It All[1]

At the time, she was seventy-four years old, widowed for more than ten years. Each of us, my mother, my brother, and I—both of us married with our own families—lived in a different town. After undergoing major surgery to remove some of her large intestine marked with diverticulitis, and having used up all the time permitted for recovery in an intensive nursing facility, we both believed that she could no longer manage to live by herself in her small but comfortable upstairs apartment. She had to move.[2]

Living with me and my family was out of the question, and she was opposed to the idea, proposed by my brother, that she move in with him in the small town some distance away. She didn't know anyone there, she argued. "All my friends are here, and I want to be with them, not in some place stuck with nobody I know." Still quite debilitated from the surgery, she was nevertheless persuaded to make the move to where he lived. At least, she told me, this would keep her in Texas, which she had come to love during her many years there.

"Maybe it'll be for just a while," my brother reasoned, "and after you get on your feet, well, we can talk about it then. About where you might go, okay?"

She felt, "in my bones," that this move was the last, that she would never get back to her apartment. "It's my home, I don't care what you think."

What had occurred, she really knew but wasn't yet prepared to admit, was that what had hitherto been only a "little discomfort" from joint aches had after the operation blossomed into widespread and aggressive arthritis. "I hurt in every joint I've got and in some I never knew I had." She had been to one specialist after another, even traveling to Nashville, where I then lived, to see still another specialist there. That worked no better than had all the others: everything the doctors tried was to no avail, causing instead severe side effects: "They all make my stomach act up something awful," she said. And, one, gold salts, was seriously debilitating, causing extensive shingles that lasted more than a year.

By the time the move was proposed, her arthritis had already become quite severe. But so had her emphysema, the result of heavy smoking of unfiltered cigarettes for more than forty years. It was increasingly difficult for her, as she said, to get "a decent breath," and any activity (walking, taking a bath, dressing) gradually but surely became hard labor. At times, any activity was additionally complicated by asthma attacks, some very harsh. In the midst of always-labored breathing, she grew to need more and more air conditioning in order to be even moderately comfortable. She eventually admitted that her lack of air conditioning, the two flights of stairs to her apartment, and the rest of needed activity just to keep herself in food made it necessary to rely on her son and his family for help—something she could not bring herself to ask of her friends.

An intelligent, articulate, caring, and independent person throughout her adult life, she gradually found herself withdrawn, depressed, isolated, and—horror of horrors in her own eyes—dependent on others, her treasured personal freedom all but gone. Still, at least at first, she made some friends where my brother lived, as she had done wherever she lived throughout her life. She came to enjoy the weekly bridge parties at their homes. She liked doing this, when she could manage to get there (driving was increasingly difficult), but she felt bad that she could not manage to have the group to her apartment (it was too tiny, she said), but the truth was she just couldn't get around and "do" like she would have wanted.

Though visits from me and my family were infrequent, because of my job and the long distance from Nashville, they were eagerly anticipated by us all. She found, though, that a day or perhaps two with us was just enough: she easily grew tired, became remote, and was quick to anger. In fact, she told me often, during her periods of real alertness, that she was undergoing significant mood changes, which she found personally humiliating, even appalling. "I'm just not that sort of person," she told us one day, "but that's the way I'm feeling more and more."

Times of cheerfulness, happy conversations with her friends and with us, laughter over past shared experiences, were ever more rare. More common were gripes, complaints, quarrelsomeness, and whiny spite. Her image of herself deteriorated, and she found that she had become more morose than lively, depressed rather than outgoing, bitter rather than interesting—precisely the sort of person she had long disliked. That she was becoming more reliant on my brother

and his wife—for cleaning the apartment, shopping, even cooking—
only fueled her bitterness.

Eventually, she found she could do little more than get up from
bed and sit at the end of her couch, the end directly in front of the
television. More often in later days, she simply slept on the couch
upright, since getting up was "easier said than done." Besides trouble
getting up, she could no longer turn the water faucet on or off,
couldn't tear off wrappings from the saltines that were now her
favorite food (no preparation needed), couldn't even get her apartment door open, much less the car door. Her world had effectively
shrunk to the space of her apartment, actually, to the space of that
one end of her couch.

She had always said to us that she would never want to live if she
could no longer "do for myself." Fiercely independent her whole life,
prizing being "beholden to nobody," she now found herself facing
what was for her the worst of all possible fates: a nursing home.
"They won't let me keep my things," she was often heard to complain when the idea came up, "and there'll be no time for myself *by*
myself and doing what *I* want to do." And, if that didn't get my
brother off the topic, he told me that she would bluster about how
"everything is run like a machine and one that doesn't work all that
well, either! You do when *they* want you to do, eat when *they* want
you to eat, everything is done for *them*, not the people there!"

The talk of a nursing home had come about because the one time
she had tried to live with my brother was an unmitigated disaster, for
everyone. She was becoming more "an old crone," she admitted, than
the lovely, lively, likeable grandmother she and we had often pic-
tured. Family life, even the minor events of daily life, were unsettled
and unsettling. With the deep love between her and my brother liter-
ally on the line, they reached the dreadful decision to move her into a
nursing home—that awful place, symbol of loss and abandonment.

But the local nursing home had no space, nor a hospital in the
likely event that she might need to be hospitalized. Her increasingly
failing pulmonary function, the arthritis, worsening asthma and
ulcers, and her dependence on numerous medications and drugs
effectively made the decision for them: she would have to be placed
in a home more than thirty miles away, in San Antonio, at least until
a place became available locally. This seemed the best of the bad
alternatives. She needed not only to eat regularly and more substan-
tially (her beloved saltines and milk had become almost the only sta-
ple), not only to have her medications controlled (she often forgot

which, whether, and when and, hence, was in effect abusing and mis-using), not only to be helped in daily needs, but also to be close to medical assistance in the event of an emergency (upper respiratory failure or infection was most feared, with her poor lungs).

By this time—"the proverbial straw," my brother said when we talked by telephone—her breathing was so shallow and feeble that she was taking in her own exhaled air and had to be placed on a portable oxygen unit even for transport to the nursing home, where she was temporarily intubated until she became a bit stronger and was taking in more oxygen. It was also necessary for her to use a wheelchair whenever she went out, which was infrequent; she could barely manage to move it by herself, and nurses were, she said, "just too busy" to come by and help. Almost completely bedridden, she was taken to the dreaded place, even more dreaded for its distance from my brother's house.

At the nursing home (assisted living facilities were practically unheard of at the time, and money was an issue), though her physical condition improved somewhat (she was extubated the day after she arrived, but remained on the portable unit), she continued to deteri-orate in mood and activity, and her few moments of real lucidity were times when she repeatedly, weepingly, declared to anyone who would listen that she saw no reason to continue to live. Her lungs were almost, and irreversibly, gone; her every joint hurt horribly; her limbs had become terribly misshapen and (to her) ugly; her proud independence seemed utterly gone and as irrecoverable as her breathing. She had no friends anywhere close by, my family and I lived more than a thousand miles away, and she was separated even from my brother and his family. "This is such a farce," she told one nurse. "Why keep up the pretense?"

She was most deeply depressed, her words recalled for us by one of the doctors who saw her there, because she had become "the very sort of person I've always despised, and I can't seem to help it. I hurt, awfully, all the time, and I can't get a decent breath. I have nothing to look forward to, can't get out of this loathsome place, I can't even walk to the bathroom without awful pain, and can only barely get my fingers to turn on the TV. Why keep it up?" I don't know what if anything the doctor said to her; he merely mentioned this conversa-tion to my brother during a visit—much the same words, he told me, she was been using while still in her little apartment close by.

Earlier in her life, she had presided over her own mother's grad-ual, painful death from cancer many years before, and she had watched her father angrily fade away from a more recent stroke, knowing all along her helplessness to stop, to help, almost even to comfort either of them. She and my father had divorced while I was still in high school, my brother then in a brief tour with the Army. But after my own tour in Korea, she and I moved in together, when I started college in another city. She had managed to survive and even heal herself from years of incapacitating alcoholism after remarrying a man who, at his best, could be described only as ineffective and pathetic. After a time free from alcohol, she then married a third time, to a man who turned out to be "as mean as a snake and closed-minded to boot," we all knew well, and whose creeping death from emphysema my mother tended daily at their home until the end. She knew full well what was in store for her.

Now, here she was, in the same condition plus other complications from arthritis, in the very condition she had solemnly sworn never to be caught up in. While dying was dreaded, death seemed a blessing, for it would bring not only relief from constant, excruciating pain, constant laboring for every breath, but, far more, relief from her having become "such a burden and trial" to her sons and their families. "This," she told her nurse one day—sufficiently impressed by it to make a note of it in her chart—"is simply intolerable, just unbearable."

We found out what had happened when, one morning, she was found comatose, barely breathing. The nurse on duty quickly put everything in motion: she called an ambulance, established temporary pulmonary assist, and sent her to the nearby hospital emergency room. She then called my brother. By the time he traveled the thirty or so miles to the hospital, she was already in the intensive care unit and still comatose. Shocked and dismayed, he had never seen anything like this before. He later told me that it was "just like one of those TV shows, just so unreal." He waited outside the ICU for some word, grief stricken and utterly unsure and in dread of what he felt would soon happen: his mother would come awake. She did, soon after, but when he got in to see her, he was met with anger, bewilderment, frustration, pleading. Unable to talk because she remained intubated, she stayed in the ICU for several days before she was stabilized and able to be extubated.

At that point, she was, he told me, "just like her old self, the one I hadn't seen in a long, long time!" But this was just for a short time, for there was still the ominous presence of the medical armamentarium. She found her voice, though, still harsh and clearly hurting from the tube that had been down her throat, but she was very, very clear: "I will never be hooked up like that again, and you better tell that nurse, that doctor, whoever did this to me, that I won't tolerate it again, never again, never! I don't want those damned machines anywhere near me, ever!"

He was, to say the least, taken aback, for he had hardly ever seen her in this sort of temper. He managed to tell her he'd do what he could. Shortly after, she was discharged back to the nursing home, where she remained for only a day or so, because in the meantime my brother had been able to find a place for her close to his home. I had flown in, and together we visited with her personal physician so that she could make her wishes "clear as a bell ringing in dead winter." After some discussion they reached an agreement to sign, jointly, the state's newly enacted directive to physicians, instructing them not to use any "mechanical or other 'artificial methods'" that would serve merely to prolong her dying and pointlessly postpone the moment of her death—this notion was quite new at that time, but we were all in agreement.

Her physician was authorized to withhold or withdraw all "life-sustaining procedures" whenever it was additionally determined by him and another licensed physician that death is "imminent," regardless of whether such procedures are utilized. A copy was placed in her medical file at the nursing home, another her doctor put in her medical file he kept in his office, and copies were given to my brother and me. Signed, sealed, delivered. So everyone believed.

Her condition, although somewhat stable, nevertheless continued to deteriorate slowly. She was encouraged to do modest exercises and to walk a bit in order to try and regain some muscle tone (lost by her recent hospitalization), but she often refused to do any. She continued to feel low, and her bitter, whiny complaining worsened.

About three months into her stay at the local nursing home, she made the effort to get up and walk to her small bathroom, but slipped and fell, breaking her hip (osteoporosis had in the meantime become generalized). She was taken to the hospital in the nearby urban center for surgical replacement of the hip joint. The surgery was, she later told my brother, "remarkable; I actually hurt less and I can even walk a bit!"

This more positive mood lasted only a few days, however, and by the time I was able to fly down and visit, she had again become bitter, morose, and angry. "I'd just as soon die, get it over with, stop this hurting," she told me. In an effort to help lighten her mood, I brought out the brand-new tape recorder I'd just bought for her. "Now you can talk to me on tape," I said, "and then send the tape to me. I'll listen, use the same tape to talk back to you, and you can then listen to me here. Voice is a lot better than handwriting, anyway," I pointed out, noting my lousy letter-writing record.

She said she'd try, "But I'm not sure I can even push that button there," she complained.

"Don't worry," I said, "I've talked with the nurses, and all you have to do is ask, and one of them will be happy to come down and do it for you."

"Ha!" her voice sarcastic and whiny, she angrily complained. "They're never here when you need them. Where were they when I broke my hip? I was on the floor more than an hour before anyone showed up!"

"It couldn't have been that long," I insisted. "I was told they got to you right away."

"That's as may be, but I can tell you a thing or two about all that . . ."

"What's that supposed to mean, Mom? Come on, all you have to do is push that button and start talking. You don't even have to get anyone else here to help; just push and talk, push and talk, okay?"

"Well, we'll see about that, won't we," she jeeringly retorted. "Just push and talk, huh? We'll see, we'll just see, what with you ready to rush on back to Nashville, getting out of here, don't know as I blame you, though, but there you'll go, and here I'll be, wasting away, lying here, fade out for old Mom, right? Just might as well disappear, just out, gone, good-bye . . ."

She fell into what seemed to us a kind of stupor. "She does that, you know," my brother said, sadness marking his voice, his shoulders drooping, hands hanging by his side, useless as his words to bring her back. "Just fades out, sort of, and you find yourself talking to the air."

"Well," I responded, "maybe she'll give it a try, you know, send me a tape or two. Maybe when she hears my talking to her, things will change, maybe. You think?"

"Just not sure, little brother, just not sure. Sometimes, she hardly seems to be there, just not there, somewhere else."

"What do you mean?"

"Well, like I said, I'll be here and her over there on that couch, and I'll maybe ask if she wants to come with me to get some tacos, or an ice cream, something anyway. But it'll be like she wasn't there, didn't hear me, and I'll have to repeat it, you know, and repeat it several times."

In fact, she made only one tape, and didn't send it. It's not clear that she remembered even talking into the recorder, for she became gradually more and more forgetful. Along with that, she was rarely alert enough to appraise herself, to realize what was happening. She became known among the home's staff, especially because of her nightly complaints, as a whiner and griper.

Then, early one morning about five months after the hip replacement, when I just got back from my morning jog, I was met with my wife's anxious eyes, her voice raveled with concern. "Your brother just called. Mom's had another. She's back in the emergency room."

"What happened?"

"I'm not sure, 'cause he was so shaken, calling from the hospital, he said Mom's been taken back."

"But why, for heaven's sake? What's gone on? When did she do it?"

"I'm trying to tell you that I don't know, only that he's really shook up, and Mom's there. It must have happened real early, 'cause it's only 7:00 right now. Sounds like the last time, you know, when they found her without her oxygen on and they took her to the ER."

"Oh, my god, she's pulled it out, I know it! She's pulled it out and now she's . . ." I couldn't quite bring myself to say it. Instead, I sat down and began to make plans, my way of avoiding the awful: call the airlines, eat breakfast, shower, shave, another cup of coffee. I flew out later that same day, full of dread about what I'd find.

Earlier that same morning, I later learned, the nurse on night duty had come by to check on my mother. For the first time in a long while, she had not been heard from in more than three hours. It was about 4 A.M. when the nurse got to her room. She found my mother comatose with shallow and infrequent breathing. The portable oxygenator's regulator was turned way down, almost to the off position.

Alarmed, the nurse immediately adjusted the regulator, called her supervisor, alerted the staff, called the local EMS, called the doctor (he was out of town), and then awaited the emergency techs. When they arrived, she was still in a deep coma, though her breathing was normalizing; they gently picked her up, put her on the stretcher, carried her out to the waiting ambulance, and took her off to the hospital thirty miles away.

"You'd better get in touch with the family," the techs said as they were about to drive off.

At this point, my brother was called, told what had happened and told to go to the hospital. "Decisions may have to be made, you know," she advised him.

"What decisions?" he blurted out, fearing the worst. "What am I supposed to do?"

"You'll need to find out what the doctors there think, then you'll know more what needs to be done. Don't worry, you'll be okay, and I'm sure your mother will be, too," she concluded, ringing off.

"You'd better take that directive thing," his wife shouted to him as he started to drive off.

"Oh, my God, do you think it's that serious?"

"You never know. Anyway, better to be safe than sorry."

He rushed back in, found the copy of the advance directive, and drove off to the hospital, arriving there not too long after the EMS techs. He was then told by the nurse at the ER admissions desk that physicians were trying to stabilize his mother's condition. She would die if they could not stabilize her. "Now," she said, far too calmly, he thought, "if you'll just complete these forms . . ."

"What? Forms? Are you out of your mind? That's my mother in there, and you want me to fill out forms?"

"Sir, we need this information in order to continue treating your mother. And you can't go back there just yet. When he can, the doctor will come out and talk with you."

"Well, what do I do with this?" sticking out his arm, the AD in hand, and he noted it was trembling as if there were a miniature tunnel of wind focused just on his hand.

"What is that?"

"It's the advance directive thing my mom filled out with her doctors about five, six months ago. We were told to bring it in to her doctors anytime she came back to the hospital. So, here," handing it to her.

"Well, I'm sure I don't know just what to do with that," she said.

"Give it to her doctor when he comes out."

"Maybe you'd best do that," she advised, and she turned back to answer the phone ringing insistently on another desk nearby.

"*Me? I* should give it to him? Doesn't anybody here know what to do with these? What the hell good are they, anyway? Aren't you people supposed to know about these things, what to do with them? Isn't it . . ."

"Sir, I'm sorry, but I really think you should just sit down, over there, and wait until the doctor comes in. I'm sure he'll know what to do. That's right, just there will be just fine. The doctor will be out shortly."

Obviously, this was at a time well before hospital personnel had much real experience with such documents. Even though the legislature in Texas had enacted the bill enabling advance directives and made them in fact legally binding, few health professionals knew about them much, less what to do with them in that rare event that one actually showed up.

Nor had many citizens much experience or understanding of them. So, my brother sat down, flipping the AD nervously, but keeping it as neat as he could. He just knew that someone, the doctor maybe, would know what he should do with it. Why in the world had his brother made such a noise about having Mom sign it anyway?

But even her own doctor back in Boerne hadn't objected, just cosigned it and put it away in her file. But now, neither of them was here, and he was, and he didn't know what exactly to do with it.

Just as he was thinking maybe he should take it back to his car, out came a white-gowned man, middle aged, with the sort of firm, positive stride and look that only a doctor could wear in this place. The brother immediately grew even more nervous, for the man looked serious, even grim. Things didn't look at all good.

It was the doctor who had been treating our mother. He told my brother that they were still trying to stabilize her, but he felt certain that would be accomplished shortly. "Then," he started to say, but was interrupted.

"Here," my brother came out with the AD, waving it in the air in front of the doctor.

"What in the . . ."

"It's the thing, the docu-, the advance directive, my mother signed," he exclaimed.

"The *what?*"

"The advance directive, you know, the thing we're supposed . . ."

"'Supposed'? 'Advance what'?" The doctor was obviously disturbed by the sight of this man standing there in his ER, standing there waving some sort of document that in fact looked rather legal, and was trying to hand it to him. What was he supposed to do with that? *What's going on here?* he muttered to himself, backing off a bit.

What's going on here? my brother mumbled to himself, stepping forward a bit, trying to give the AD to the doctor, who kept backing off.

The nurse found that moment to come out of the door to the ER rooms, and cried out, "What's going on here? Doctor, is this man threatening you? Sir, back off now, easy does it, just back away and nobody'll get hurt."

"Get hurt? Ma'am, I'm just trying to give this thing, this advance directive, to the doctor, like I was told I was supposed to."

"The what?" she was almost shouting.

"Look here," the doctor felt things were getting out of hand, and wanted to take control. "Look here, what is that, that 'advance directive'?"

"I thought you'd know; I was told you'd know, and that I should give it to you."

"I don't understand, I'm afraid. Why give it to me?"

"'Cause it says, it says right there, what my Mom wants and doesn't want."

"Oh, wait a minute," the nurse chimed in, "I know what that is." Turning to the doctor, she explained, "You remember, last year when the legislature passed that bill? The one that lets people tell us what they want to have done or not done when they're terminally ill?"

"Oh, that thing," the doctor said, obviously relieved he was no longer being pressed back by my brother, yet disturbed at this turn of events. "But the lady, your mother . . . look, let me explain here. We've already put her on the ventilator, she wasn't breathing at all well, so we put her on the vent, the ventilator, and once that's been done, well, we did it to stabilize her, like I said from the beginning . . ."

"Is she not going to make it this time?" the brother blurted out.

"Would we put her on the vent, intubate and everything, if she was dead?" the doctor couldn't help himself.

"I don't know, all I know is I'm supposed to give you this," and he tried again to hand it over to the doctor.

He, however, wanted no part of it, and backed off again, declaring as he was about to get out of there, "I mean, she's already on the vent, and we can't take her off of that, we can't kill her, don't you know, and if you want to kill her, well, you can just go in there and do it yourself, 'cause I'm sure as hell not going to kill her. If you want that, that's your choice, but I'll have no part of it. None. We've already put her on life-saving equipment, and these cannot be removed. If you'd gotten in here earlier, before we did that, well, maybe we wouldn't have put it all on. But it's there now, and I'm sure not going to take it off."

"Yes," the nurse came in, "and we'll have to evaluate her after a bit, find out just what's happened, then, when we know that, we'll have to transfer her to the ICU for further evaluation and such. Until we know all that, well, as I understand it, that directive just isn't appropriate. Okay?"

And with that, he took off, muttering to himself still, and leaving in his wake my brother, clearly disturbed by that speech, by the very idea that this, this directive, made him look like he wanted to kill his own mother, *him*, who had loved her all his life, who had taken her in.

The nurse took his arm gently and led him back to a chair. "Easy, sir, you should just sit down a moment. You're obviously not feeling well. Please, just try and ignore what the doctor just said. I know he didn't mean that, and anyway, we've never had this sort of document presented to us before. We really don't know quite what to do with it. But, if you'll just hang onto it for a bit, I'll try and find someone who knows about these things. That's right, just sit back. Would you like a sedative? Something to help you relax? No? Well, how about some coffee?"

He allowed himself to be led out into a hallway, down a bit into a room with a pot of coffee, and took the cup she offered him, then walked back with her to the waiting room, sat down, sipped, thought, folded up the directive and slipped into his shirt pocket.

"Is there anyone you would like to telephone?" she asked. "I must get back inside, but if you'd like to call someone, just ask the lady over there at the desk." And, with that, she made her way out of the door leading back to where his mother, his own mother, was lying, near death he was convinced, all plugged and hooked up to this and that sort of instrument, but dying all the same.

Then he remembered his brother, me. *Oh*, he murmured to himself, *I'd best get him on the line and let him know what's happening.* With that, he walked over to the lady, asked to use a phone, was directed back out into the hallway, where he found a pay phone, dug in his pocket, and luckily found a quarter. He dialed and waited. *Damn*, he said to himself, *it's still only 7 o'clock; I bet little brother isn't even awake yet. Hate to wake him up with this, but got to do it. Come on, answer the phone, little brother, answer the phone.*

I was not in. My wife was, and he tried to explain to her how things were, there in the ER with that doctor and what he said. He was clearly still emotionally distraught, still bleary from the abrupt awakening, stunned from what he had seen and heard in the ER. Later, when I talked with him, he had to confess that, no, he hadn't really read the damned thing, didn't know that the doctor's words about not being able to remove life supports after they were in place was not at all true. He was clear, though, that Mom did not want "those blasted machines" again, but he was not clear just when that "wish" would or could prevail. He managed to point out that the doctors, and that nurse, had (after he had thought about the confrontation, no other word for it) stressed that they were not able yet to determine whenever death "was imminent," so they "had to run those tests, didn't they?"

I had in fact read the directive. Not only had I read it, I had prepared one for myself, my wife, and my adult children. I knew the doctors were wrong, that they probably had never even cast an eye on any directive, and were also probably both angry and anxious about seeing the piece of paper. It wasn't difficult to envision the scene or to imagine how my brother was feeling.

I couldn't figure out, though, how serious my mother's condition was at that moment. There was not enough information from my brother, not enough from the doctors, not enough from anyone or anywhere. Having been involved in many such situations in my work, however, I suspected that the scene in the ER with my brother amounted to little more than the strong-arm tactics of a self-confident trauma physician who was additionally pissed at having to face such a situation, one he had little real understanding of and no experience with.

So, okay, I mused to myself while the plane was already well on its way to where I knew I should have already been, *what we have here is a failure to communicate*—disturbed, yet amused at the cliché, for it seemed true enough, after all, even if it didn't help at all figure out where the fault, if any, lay, much less what needed to be done.

Soon after I arrived that afternoon, I tried to find my brother but was told he had left. "I guess he went home, for there's nothing either of you can do at this point," I was told by the admissions clerk in the ER. I then asked to see the physician who had taken care of my mother and had talked with my brother. By that time, however, they had already determined enough to have my mother transferred to the ICU, up on the seventh floor. Calling my brother, I learned nothing new, only that he had been told to go on home until.

"Until what?"

"Well, I guess until they can figure out what's happened."

"They don't know?"

"Not from what they told me, and anyway, she's pretty heavily sedated, they said, and we've got to wait until that wears off."

"Well, I'm going to try to find someone who'll talk to me," I said, "I'll call you later when I get ready to come out, though I'm thinking of staying close by in some motel."

"Don't do that. Just come on out. We're not far and can get in right away if we have to. Besides, we've got a nice place for you to relax, get some sleep, and have a good meal."

"I'll let you know later, but you're probably right."

Some of the key pieces gradually fell into place. I learned from the ICU charge nurse that Mom was "resting quietly" and that, "no, there was no determination," at least not as yet about whether she was "terminal." The nurse seemed distinctly uncomfortable when I raised the issue, clearly not wanting to discuss the matter with me.

"You'll have to talk with the doctor about that," she said.

She did, however, let me see Mom briefly. When I went in to the cubicle, I confronted a sight I had desperately hoped I would never see, my mother like this, comatose, plugged in, intubated, the works. *Good lord*, I thought. *What happened for things to come to this?*

Going back to the nursing station, I asked her if I could see Dr. Reyes—a pulmonary specialist who had seen Mom several times before, including when she was in the nursing home down the street.

I assumed that this doctor was in charge and had at least stopped by to see my mother. She said she knew Dr. Reyes but that he had not seen my mother, for he was out of town when the "incident," as she called it, occurred. Dr. Reyes' patients were being seen by his partner, Dr. Gaylord.

Not only was this doctor unacquainted with Mom and her condition, but a quick call to my brother made it clear that Mom had never seen Dr. Gaylord, much less been treated by him. "Anyway," I told him, "the ones that saw her were those in the ER. I don't know how they arrange such things here, do you?"

"Not really. Of course, they probably have a physician on staff who sees all ICU patients, but I'm not sure whether her doctor in San Antonio—the one who treated her lung condition—or the one here locally will check on her."

"Well, I'll do what I can to find out who's supposed to diagnose and take care of her, okay?"

"Yeah, good luck on that."

"I'll let you know if I find out anything. And, I'll come on out to your house as soon as I do find out something."

But though Gaylord had come by for a brief visit, he was no longer at the hospital. Having already completed his rounds, he was on his way back to his office. I then asked the nurse for his office number so I could call him. She dialed on her phone and let me have it as it was ringing. Stepping aside, as far as the cord would allow, I managed to get through to Dr. Gaylord, as his nurse was apparently put on notice of my impending arrival.

I learned little, however, only that Dr. Gaylord had in fact seen her after her admission to the ICU but that, although he was listed as the physician "in charge," he was not the physician with whom I needed to talk—especially about "removal of life supports, which is probably not appropriate," I was told, "at this time, not as I understand what Dr. Evans, the ICU physician on staff there, told me this morning. He's the doctor you'll have to talk with. Your mother is still heavily sedated, and until that wears off it just isn't possible to determine the extent of the damage, if any, she suffered."

"Well, okay, but where is this Dr. Evans? I obviously have to talk with him."

"You should be able to get to him there, since he pretty much stays close by the ICU. I think he has an office right around the corner from the nursing desk, in fact. Ask the nurse to show you."

Which I did. And I actually found Dr. Evans. As I had suspected, however, communication was at best very difficult, made positively awkward at the first mention of advance directives. On showing Dr. Evans my own copy of the advance directive, I was told I shouldn't be in such a hurry. Evans said he fully understood the directive. "You know," he pointed out, "we're beginning to see more of those, but mainly here in the ICU, hardly ever in the ER or on the floor." He was in fact, he declared, willing to comply with his mother's expressed and written wishes. He could do this, however, he said, "only after I'm satisfied that in my medical judgment her condition is truly irreversible and terminal," the very words of the directive, of course.

Evans pointed out, though, that her condition was currently masked by the sedatives. What neurological tests were done, in the ER, he reported, had thus far showed some, but only slight, telltale signs of numerous, frequent, tiny seizures. The "appropriate response"—a phrase Evans was very fond of—to these came in the form of medications designed to lessen the chances of their continuing to occur.

"Unfortunately," he went on, "the medication we have to use also tends to mute neurologic activity generally." Thus, he was unable "to determine whether there had been brain damage"—the first time the phrase with its dreaded words had come up, and, despite much experience with such phrases in the course of my work, I shuddered inwardly at its sound—"from the hypoxic incident, much less the extent of it or whether recovery of some brain function is still possible." For these determinations, Evans told me, more time was needed.

"How much time?"

"Well, as I said, we shouldn't be in any hurry here."

"I'm not in a 'hurry,' as you put it, not at all. I merely want to know how much time you need before you can tell more about her condition, her prospects, whether she'll ever recover or will be left just a vegetable."

"I don't approve of that sort of language," Evans was clearly growing impatient.

"Well, what words would you use for extensive brain damage?"

"We don't yet know just how extensive it is," Evans replied with an edge.

Which I picked up on immediately. "You mean there *has* been brain damage, you just don't know how much?"

"Well, sure, yes, I mean, yes, there surely has been some brain damage . . ."

"And why didn't you tell my brother about this when he was here earlier? When we talked, he never mentioned 'brain damage.'"

"Well, I had only a brief moment with him, right after your mother was brought up here. Plus, he was clearly distraught and seemed anxious to be somewhere else, to leave things to us. Look, I have other patients I must see, and we can't do any more at this time anyway . . ."

"Are you a neurologist?" I asked, rather more bluntly than I had intended, but I refused to give up or get out of the way.

"Why, no, my field is pulmonology, like most of us directors of ICU's . . ."

"Then, how do you know whether or how extensive there has been brain damage? Has she been seen by a neurologist yet?"

"No, not yet. Now look, I really must get on with my patients. I just don't have time for this sort of thing. I will ask the nurse to chat with you, if you want, and perhaps we can talk later."

With that, Dr. Evans took off down the hall.

The ICU nurse could add nothing of import so I went back into the cubicle to be with Mom. But all I could know for sure from looking at her was that regular, ventilator-induced up-and-down of her frail chest. The monitors told me little, just that vital signs of vital systems were showing that things were working, or were being made to work by all the "stuff" hooked up to her.

I realized, too, that it was pointless for me to stay there. I was helpless, at the mercy of that Dr. Evans, who was clearly unwilling to do more than wait and make us wait, too.

After spending the night with my brother, and talking things over as much as we could, we decided that I would return and try to get hold of her main doctor, the one who was substituting for her regular one. We realized that even that doctor was nothing like her "regular doc," my brother emphasized, "it's just that when she goes to that hospital, her doc here, Dr. Montgomery, never goes over there to see her. It's like he can't or won't take over when Mom's over there. And anyway, he's somewhere on vacation right now."

"Well, let me go on in and give that one doctor, Dr. Gaylord, a call. See what's going on this morning. Man! I'm really bushed!"

"The plane and everything, right?"

"The plane and, yeah, *every*thing. I really don't know what to expect, you know. We won't know anything until, and if, she comes out of that coma. I just don't think it's all because of the drugs she's on. I think there has been some brain damage, has to be! That guy in the ICU, Dr. Evans, you know he said as much when I asked, point blank. He admitted it, but I don't think he wanted to. Just can't figure, you know, why the hell they don't want to tell us anything. Anyway . . ." My voice trailed off.

"Well, let me know, okay? I still have that trip out West I should take, I should say I got scheduled already."

"So, go ahead, take it. I'll see to things. Heaven knows, you've had to take care of things since Mom moved down here."

"Well, okay, then, just call if you learn anything, alright?"

"Yeah, well, I'd best be on my way. What's the time?

"Almost 7. It'll take you maybe thirty minutes, forty-five at the outside, to get there, and someone should be there by then, don't you think?"

"It's Sunday, you know."

"Does that make a difference?"

"Well, I don't know, don't know how they run things at this hospital. Anyway, then, I'll be off. Appreciate the loan of the car."

"Least I can do."

After getting Gaylord's phone number and trying it, without success, before I left, I took my brother's car and drove to the hospital. When I got there, I placed another call, managed, wonder of wonders, to get Gaylord on the line, introduced myself again, and, as I had expected, found out only that he had nothing new for me; however, Gaylord, admitting that he was still "in charge of her case," said he'd be out before too long and would meet with me.

Immediately after breakfast at the cafeteria, I went back to the ICU, to see Mom. No change. Still nothing like alertness. *Coma, comatose, in a coma, torpid, inert*—I had to make a deliberate effort to stop the litany. My eye on the heart monitor's zig and zag, up and down, the beat regular, lights blinking, a beep quietly beeping—I left, couldn't stay there, went out to the waiting room, but before I could sit, in walked Dr. Gaylord, with Dr. Evans at his side.

Dr. Evans, though, took the lead, with Gaylord standing to the side. Evans was brisk, though friendly, restating what he had already stated the day before and noting that there had been no change since then, except that the "little seizures" were no longer occurring. He had, thus, been able to stop the medications—"You concur, Jack?" he asked.

"Of course," Gaylord promptly replied.

"Well, then, I think we're on track. We can do the appropriate tests in about twenty-four hours. In the meantime . . ."

"Whoa, wait a minute. Can I ask a question?"

"Of course, what is it?"

"I asked you the last time we talked whether a neurologist had seen my mother, and you said that none had. I would . . ."

"That's correct, and as I mentioned then, I see no need for that at this time."

"Well, I do," I was getting a bit agitated. "I want to know what sort of brain damage there's been, and I think it's only proper to ask for a neurologist to see Mom with that in mind."

"Well, we could of course do that, normally, but at this time, there's only, I think, one consulting neurologist on call, and I don't think she's available."

Dr. Gaylord stepped in, sensing that I might be getting a bit angry. "Why don't you let me handle that, Dr. Evans? I know the neurologist you have in mind, and . . ."

"Well, if that's the way you want it, I'll just let you take over."

"Can I get a word in here?" They stopped, and turned to me. "I'm not trying to cause any problems. I should tell you that I work in a health care setting, in fact at Vanderbilt University Medical Center, and . . ."

"Oh, are you a doctor?"

"Not the kind you probably mean," I replied. "I helped her fill out that advance directive some months ago, along with her local doctor and my brother. I know something about these things, 'cause I've been in medical ethics for a long time, and . . ."

Before I could go any further, Dr. Evans erupted. Swift, harsh words poured out. "Ethics? What's that supposed to mean? You think we're being unethical here? Well, let me tell you straight and clear: there are no ethical problems here, none, zero. The only questions are medical and legal. I am the physician of record here and nothing gets done about that living will thing until I say it gets done. You understand? I want that perfectly clear. And in my medical judgment, until I can do the right tests, I can't say that she's incurable or terminable or whatever, not yet, by no means."

"But if there has been brain damage, like you said last night, then she might be not only irreversible but, in a neurologist's judgment also terminal, and if so, the directive is legally binding."

"No way," Evans replied, "not unless and until I am clear about that and then determine whether in my medical judgment she's reached that stage. And I can't do that until at least twenty-four hours, after the tests. As it is . . ."

"As it is, like I said earlier, you don't know and you not only need to do tests, it seems to me you need an expert judgment, a neurologist, to come in and see. Isn't that right?" I asked turning to Dr. Gaylord. "Aren't you her attending at this time?"

"Well, yes, I am. And, I think that what you're asking could certainly be arranged, but Dr. Evans is still the physician of record and what he says goes, I think."

"I thought you were the attending."

"Well, yes, I am, but I am not going to contravene what Dr. Evans says in any case."

"Well," I was getting angry, "I can tell you this much: ethics or law or all of them put together, or put aside completely, I think it's only proper that you set up that consult and that you do it today, as soon as it can be done. That's what I think, and to put a cap on it, I should also point out that I am my mother's attorney-in-fact, I am listed on her durable power of attorney for healthcare decisions, and until and if she can do it herself, my word counts as being as good as hers. And I want a neurologist to look at her."

"Set it up, Jack, would you? I'm outta here," Evans quickly turned away.

As he started to walk off, he was stopped in the hallway by my brother, who had been standing there for some time. Realizing that Evans appeared angry, my brother kept his cool and urged Evans to remain calm. Why, he wanted to know, was twenty-four hours all that important? Evans' reply was indeed couched in anger.

"I will tell you this: if you had not agreed with the ER doctor yesterday morning, if you'd demanded that no vent be put in place, well, then, we'd not be having this talk right now. I gather you did agree to that, however, and this means we can't remove those supports until things are a good deal clearer than they are right now. I must be medically certain before I ever do that sort of thing."

At which point I stepped up, with the idea of trying to let this doctor know how harsh that ER doc had been and that, far from any agreement, my brother had in fact been bullied, and in any case Mom had already been intubated by the time my brother had arrived. But, I couldn't get to the words before Dr. Evans huffed off down the hallway.

So I turned to Dr. Gaylord, still standing there looking somewhat nonplussed. "Dr. Gaylord, my brother and I want you to have a neurologist look at our mom. It seems to me reasonably clear, from what Dr. Evans stated last night, that serious brain damage has in fact occurred and that the coma is permanent. Mom isn't going to come out of that. The only question is how much brain damage, and I know what my mother would want: if she can't be brought back to the point she was at before all this happened, well, she just wouldn't want to keep on living. Am I right?" he turned to my brother.

"That's what Mom said, more'n once, too."

Dr. Gaylord agreed and immediately went to the ICU desk and called for the consult. As it turned out—*the first fortunate thing that's happened*, I thought to himself—a Dr. Maureen Braun was not only available, but was actually in the hospital and—*wonder of wonders*, I mused—willing to come down within a short time.

Which she did, arriving just after my brother had left the hospital. They had thought that nothing would be known for at least twenty-four hours, so he could go ahead with his trip. So, I was by myself, a bit unnerved by the rapid appearance of the neurologist and whatever she might find. I stood waiting at the ICU nursing desk for the neurologist to complete her examination. Should I try to find my brother? His wife? I decided not, not before I learned what the neurologist had to say.

Dr. Braun came out more quickly than I expected. She confirmed my feeling, though, that Mom had indeed suffered quite severe brain damage. She wanted to make sure of her examination, first, however, by having another EEG performed by the technician, so she turned to the nurse on duty and asked that the tech be brought in as soon as possible and then turned back to me. "I understand that your mother was on oxygen at the nursing home?"

"Yes, that's right."

"Well, she has, I think, suffered a pretty severe stroke, which probably is what brought her in here in the first place. While here, as is noted in her medical chart, she's had frequent, though less severe, strokes. All this combined means that there has doubtless been considerable brain damage, and it is no doubt irreversible. The coma she's in right now, you could say, is no doubt permanent. She'll not come out of it."

"And, does this mean that she's incurable?"

"I'd say so. If you are referring to the language of the directive to physicians?"

"Well, actually, I wasn't right then, but, sure, why not?"

"If the EEG tech verifies what I believe will be found, then, yes, she is 'incurable' and 'terminal.' She won't recover from the coma. From all I can tell at this time, she probably has no more than 25 percent brain capacity left, if that much."

"My lord, that's awful, I, I . . ."

"I know, I know, and I'm terribly sorry to appear so blunt about it. In any case, let me get the tech here, and we'll see about things."

"Yes, yes, by all means." I was beginning to feel what I hadn't felt since flying down here. My *mother*, *my* mother, was all but dead—and memories and unexpected feelings came pouring in.

About two hours later, Dr. Braun returned to find me sitting in the ICU waiting room. Her visit was brief and admirably to the point.

"Your mother has in fact suffered considerable brain damage, as I suspected this morning. The EEG confirms that the coma is profound and permanent."

I didn't say anything, so Dr. Braun continued.

"I'm terribly sorry to have to be the one to tell you this. Your mother has suffered massive brain and brain-stem damage. I believe it is not only permissible to have the ventilator removed, but positively required that it be done. It is providing no benefit whatever."

I was still silent, only nodding as the neurologist spoke.

"Well, okay, then, if it is alright with you, I'll have the nurse get Dr. Evans—have you met him yet?" Seeing my nod, she continued, "It's Dr. Evans' place to do this, so I'll have him paged. Again, I'm sorry, very sorry to be the one to tell you all this, but in my judgment this is the right thing to do."

"Believe me, Dr. Braun, I sincerely appreciate your being so honest about it, telling it just like it is. That's all I've wanted all along."

"I think I know that."

"Well, well, so what should I do in the meantime?"

"Would you like to be with your mother while the ventilator is removed?"

"Let me think about that, okay? I think so, but let me think about it. I've dealt with many such situations at Vanderbilt, but this is different, you know? Now, it's my mother . . ."

"That's fine. I'll talk with the nurse now. I don't think I'll be seeing you, so I'll just say goodbye now."

"Dr. Braun?" I called out before she could move away.

"Yes?"

"Dr. Braun, thank you, thank you so much, for what you've done. It's made it all much clearer, no matter how hard, it's at least much clearer."

"Thanks for that. . ."

"But I do have another question."

"What is it?"

"Well, this isn't easy, you know? But I wanted to know, about something you said earlier, about Mom's having had a severe stroke while she was still at the nursing home?"

"Yes, I recall. She must have had a really severe stroke, one that initiated all the subsequent events."

"Yes, well, I understand, you see, and just wondered, you see, it crossed my mind and I didn't know what to think . . ."

"Why don't you just come on out and say what's on your mind?"

"Well, yeah, sure. You see, I just wondered whether she could have had that sort of stroke while she was still on oxygen, or whether all the damage and such happened after, maybe even because, she was off . . ."

"I'm not sure I understand: do you mean to say that she was not on oxygen at the nursing home?"

"No, she was, only the nurse there said she found Mom with her portable unit turned off and the, what do you call them? The prongs? The prongs were not in place, not wrapped around her ears, you know? like they were taken off or something . . ."

"Well, that's news. Could she have suffered this brain damage by not having an adequate oxygen supply, because that's what it would be. Do you know why she was not on the prongs, the unit turned off?"

"No, see, and well, that was my question . . ."

"Well, I don't know about that. I can say, though that, yes, she surely could have suffered both a stroke and brain damage due to the lack of oxygen. She might, additionally, have had some damage from lack of oxygen, then, secondary to that, suffered one or more strokes. There's just no way of telling at this point, without an autopsy, just what sequence of events occurred."

"Well, we don't want any autopsy. I just needed to think about things a bit more. That's helpful, Dr. Braun, very helpful. Thanks, again."

"Yes, well, I'll be off now."

"Yes," I replied more to myself than to her, as she was already at the nurse's desk talking. The nurse paged Dr. Evans. Soon, I heard the nurse's phone ring. She picked it up, listened, said something, then looked at me, said something else, nodded, and hung up.

She walked over to me. Speaking softly, she told me that Dr. Evans was not able to come right then, and had asked her, the nurse, to disconnect the ventilator from my mother. "Dr. Braun said you might want to be present. Do you?"

"So, Evans isn't coming?"

"That's right, and he asked me to do the disconnect."

"Yes, I'd like to be with you for this," replied, "I'd like to be with my mother."

The ventilator was removed with the tube kept in place along with the oxygen mask. The nurse, saying that "this wouldn't take very long," returned to her station, while I stayed by Mom's side. Remarkably, before long she began spontaneous, but very irregular breathing. After this labored on for a half hour, with no detectable change, I walked back to the station, and asked if the nurse would extubate.

"I'm not sure I can do that," she replied.

"Well, my mother just keeps on breathing, no change, and none in the monitors, so far as I can tell. Why can't you extubate? Isn't that tube supposed to come out, too?"

"My orders did not include that; however, let me call Dr. Evans again, and see if that can be done."

While she called, I went back into my mother's cubicle, not a little shaken by the turn of events. Her situation was unchanged. I glanced at my watch, noting that it had now been more than forty-five minutes since the ventilator had been disconnected. Just then, the nurse returned, saying that Dr. Evans had given his permission for extubation.

"I'm not sure you want to be here for this," she said.

"Why not?"

"Well, this can get very difficult for family, for patients often show agonal breathing . . . do you know what that is?

"Yes, I think I do; she'll struggle for breath, right?"

"Yes, and that's hard to watch, always hard for anyone to watch, much less family members."

"Well, okay, I see, well, uhmm, I think I should be here, so go ahead."

"Are you sure?"

"I'm at this point not sure of anything," I said, " but yes, I'm sure, I guess. Yes, now, well, let's go."

"This isn't easy, either," she said as she made a great effort to pull out the tube. "These can get lodged, too tight . . ." Then with a sort of pop, the tube eased out, the mask left in place.

"Can you remove the mask, too, please? I'd like to see her without that mask on, if that's okay."

"Sure, I can do that." And the mask was removed.

Sitting there by her side, watching her strain and labor for each breath, her emaciated, delicate chest heaving each time as if reaching out for air. I watched, awed, trembling, my hand shaking, as Mom, or her body, struggled, clutching almost, it seemed, for a breath, then another, and another. I stared at the heart monitor as its thin tracing of each beat of her heart was marked electronically on the screen, a jiggle up and down, gradually slowing down then. She gasped, the monitor's line zigging rapidly, then slower, and slower, marking the final measure of her life, until at last, with awful certainty, her breathing ceased and that zig-zagging line edged to an agonizing, still, stunning flatness. Mom was finally, surely dead, her face—spare and gaunt and tortured even in her coma—now relaxed, at ease, reposed, and, somehow, strangely, empty.

As was I emptied of sense and sight, heard nothing, yet felt my hand on the bed cover, just over where her hand had been, was still yet seemed no longer there, merely a lump, a thing like a piece of wood. Emptied, too, or dulled, muted with not feeling anything, stock still, silent, sitting now (I don't know how I got to the chair), watching the no-longer-being-there of my mother. *Odd*, I remember thinking to myself, *how peculiar, she was just there, coma, yes, but there, now not. So, where is she? If she is there no more, then where did she go? Did she go anywhere? Cease to be? But how? What moved her breathing, her heart, her blood, her pulse, what? How? Empty, emptied, vacant, unoccupied, no longer there, blank, uninhabited: where are you, Mom?*

Cleaning up her room at the nursing home when he got back from his trip, my brother and I came across an audiotape, apparently one Mom had made with the recorder I had left.

"She did make a tape after all, see?" I said. "Why didn't she send it to me, I wonder?"

"Don't know. I just don't know. Damn, I'm sorry I wasn't there, you know, with you in the ICU when she left us."

Left us? I mumbled to myself. Aloud, I replied, "You know it's okay, it's fine. There was no need of us both being there. Just leave it, okay? Just leave it."

"Hey, don't get angry . . ."

"I'm not, not at all. Do you mind if I take the tape, see what she said? I suppose it was for me, it's what I asked her to do, right?"

"Well, well, yeah, sure, that's fine. Let me hear it sometime, okay?"

"Yeah, that's fine. I'll make a transcription or something, see that you get it anyway."

We continued cleaning up her remaining things. *So few things*, I thought to myself, *so few, and Mom loved her things, her clothes, her trinkets, her jewelry. Where are they now?*

After I returned to Nashville later that evening, I put the tape on his own recorder, sat back, coffee in reach, and listened.

The tape was made only a week prior to her second "pulmonary crisis." She is by herself, talking quietly, and after a while seems to forget that she is talking and recording for she just slips in and out of talk, long periods of silence, then she picks up and talks. She says, in part:

I know . . . [clears throat] . . . I know . . . I know now that no matter . . . no matter how long my sentence is, . . . it's gonna be spent in this nursing home, alone, nobody around, nobody to tell my troubles to . . . 's far as my family is concerned . . . [very long pause] But I'm glad they don't have to sit and watch me die. I had to sit and watch Mother die, an' it was terrible, just terrible. I think I'll spare my children that . . . not that I have any choice about it . . . Can't think of a worse sentence, no worse way to spend it th' in . . . than in a nursing home. 'Home,' hah! Some home this is. It's just like bein' in jail, really. You have no rights; you're just a number, a bed even, gets down to it. A baby. An' all the bodies are old and worn out, an' yours is no different than anybody else's. . . . An' I found out that it's not any advantage at all . . . to have your . . . brains left, because, when you question anything, they think you're trying to tell them how to run their business . . . [clears throat] . . . It's better not to question, it's better just t' go 'n accept their orders like any child would: no questions, jus' do. . . [very long pause while she apparently tries to turn off the recorder; then silence, apparently succeeding]

Later in the tape, possibly on another day (for she doesn't give the date this time), she reflects:

Well, here's *another* day . . . 's another day but not another dollar, hah! . . . I'll swear, how slowly they pass, these days . . . and you wonder why I can't be cheerful about things . . . [long pause] I'm tryin', I really am tryin', don't you know, but just not getting' anywhere, nowhere, no . . . where . . . When he [apparently referring to her pulmonary specialist, Dr. Reyes] told me that there wasn't any possible chance for me to get out and have another apartment on my own . . . and, an' . . . [wheezing] . . . that I'd always have to live here, or in a place like this . . . that, tha' . . . did something to me . . . I just couldn't shake that feeling, . . . I know . . . I'm nothing but a gloomy Gus, dismal, dark and sad, me, and all that . . . You'll just have to bear with me . . . I may get used to it, may not, just don't know . . . I may not . . . 'ts a bad deal all 'round. . .

And, still later on the same tape:

Yeah, that's me alright, just ol' gloomy Gus today for sure, I sound just like despairin' Don, don't I? . . . Well, unfortunately for everyone that's just how I feel . . . I'm gonna stop now.

Maybe I'll feel more cheerful another time, feel more like talking . . . so, well, Bye-bye.

All through the tape, her voice is slow and halting, and there are many pauses, most of them long and none of them filled with "er," "uh," or other such fillers. In part, it seems, these pauses seem due to her struggle to get "a decent breath," for her lungs were almost completely gone. Then, she has to talk with the nasal prongs in place, which seem to irritate her. And, not accustomed to talking to a recorder, her voice keeps fading away and then coming back in more strongly, though it's never very strong, for she never has much air to push out and shape into words. Her tone quality is breathy, at times raspy (again, her lungs). At times it is whiny ("I'll swear, how slowly they pass" and "you have no rights; you're just a number").

Her voice is often weepy and choked ("how long my sentence is," "watch me die," "it was terrible"). The pitch is medium, though at times her voice drops lower (rarely does it raise to a higher tone). The volume has some swings to it from dull and quiet to more lively and more shrill ("they treat you like a baby"). Her articulation is quite precise, however, even when there is some slurring (possibly in part due to her loose false teeth, the lower plate especially). Her word choice is relatively precise and simple, her sentences, even with pauses, quite easy to detect and straightforward, with little syntactic distancing (using "you" when talking about herself, e.g., with only occasional slips: "You have no rights"). Her talk seems orderly and consistent, which is striking considering what she is saying and how very poor her health.

Despite the latter, especially her poor lung capacity and consequent struggles in breathing, she presents as alert, even though profoundly sad and depressed. She understands how dependent she has become, and this reliance is a source of grief for her. She now is "fated" without her control of life she does not want. Thus, at times she seems resigned to that fate, despondent yet reaching for dignity as she talks of her death, of what being in the nursing home is doing to her. Her lament that she has become "gloomy and sad" sounds frank and is spoken with a kind of self-respect she at other times sees as damaged. She seems completely honest about herself, a bit hostile at times (about the nursing home, for instance) but not actively angry. Her moods, though at times sharply clear, are most often muted and leveled down; she is pessimistic about her present and future. Somewhat resentful at her fate, yet there are moments when she has clearly recovered the person she once was: active, spunky, alert, outgoing. Then, this quickly fades. Once tough, she has now withdrawn.

That is the story I want to tell. Not all of it, not yet. But the quick and harsh. The "harsh," for I remain in considerable guilt. I knew, as did my brother, how profoundly sad our mother had become. We knew, too, how deeply she dreaded going into the nursing home—that "prison" where she saw herself as reliant and felt trapped. And, we knew how repulsed she was by those "old bodies," all worn out; revolted, too, by her own having become one of them, no longer, she believed, the charming and attractive woman of her youth and middle years. We knew her hurt, her pain, her suffering. Yet we not only let her go into that "prison," we—certainly I, for I can and will speak only for myself, lived in a kind of careful ignorance of what had happened to her, of where she was living out her final days and in what miserable condition. That is unconscionable; that is what I must face and live with, and I mention it only to keep the reminders in place. Will I too wind up in the same sort of place in the same sort of condition? What an awful variation on Bill Cosby's famous joking "curse" on children: may they grow up to have children just like themselves.

That said, what can I make of my mother's story? She was left pretty much alone, obliged to live in a strange place and among strangers (other patients, staff). Living with other patients (all old, all "worn out"), she lived with constant, face-to-face reminders of herself as seen by them. Though she still had her "brains" left, that made little or no difference, in fact it was much, much worse: every thought, every word, every question, just rebounds back (they "think you're tryin' to tell them how to run their business"). So, she learned, as must all other patients, that it is "best" not to question, not even to talk, eventually, to the extent possible, not to think. "Just accept" and "do what you're told."

She was told by her doctor that she could never again live on her own, and this "did somethin' to me . . . I really couldn't shake it." This, we knew, came on her for a lot of reasons, but one of the most significant for her was that she had pretty much guaranteed that "fate" by the way she had lived for the prior decade. It was therefore the hardest of hard things to have to face that history, for she now understood herself as condemned to it. Most horrible was that her sons would now have to "sit and watch me die" just as she had done with her own mother (and, I should add, her own father as well as her last husband). Now she had "no choice." So, try as she might to be "cheerful" and not a "gloomy Gus," she realized that "I'm not getting anywhere with that." Realizing that serves as but another source of sadness, regret, disappointment.

Yet, and yet again: what could my brother and I have done? He had tried having her live with him, and it wound up in disaster, for both of them. Her forgetfulness (about medications, for instance) prompted the very sort of reliance she did not want; their habituated lifestyle was a constant source of complaint for her. Things became so awkward and excruciating both for the family and for her that anger and spitefulness became increasingly the marks of each day. And, in those ever more rare moments of clarity, both realized that "this has to stop." Nor would it have been any different had she tried to live with me and my family. We both had simply too many independent and ultimately conflicting histories for that to work out. Some families can do this. We could not, and eventually we all had to face it, painful as it was.

Thus, "what could be done, alternately" was extraordinarily limited. Not that any of us liked it, for each of us continually talked about "doing something different," to no avail. There is this as well: everything we knew about each other, about her especially, confirmed that she was, and remained even for much of her stay in the nursing home, an intelligent, vibrant person with a true knack for making other people feel comfortable, for being friendly and for making friends. She was never uncomfortable with strangers; to the contrary. Yet, her recent past was marked by her withdrawal from friends and casual contacts; she repeatedly said how she could no longer "get up the effort" to clean up, get dressed, and be with others. Her lungs were practically shot, and her arthritis proved unmanageable and was thus a major factor in her inability to clean and dress herself, much less to grab and turn things such as door handles, even the stove and refrigerator. By the time she finally agreed to go to the nursing home, her breathing was so severely impaired that she could hardly sustain more than a few words at a time—hence the characteristic pauses on the recording. Thanks to the arthritis, moreover, she had become an "embarrassment to myself" in appearance and conversation: her limbs deformed, her face deeply lined from years of deep pain and struggles for breath.

Embedded in all this is a history, her history, which reveals several complex and centering moral themes. The first one still rings in my ears, for she was constantly saying it: she was deeply repulsed by the very idea of having my brother and I have to "sit and watch me die," just as she had been obliged to undergo with her mother and father and, later, her husband. Painfully, with agonizing and gradual diminishment of mind, of person, of self. Seeing a person lose her wits, becoming de-mented and wit-less, this is surely among the deepest fears we all have. I surely do. She never wanted anyone she loved to have to witness that. She not only cooperated in her placement in the nursing home; in many ways, she positively sought it. I know the paradox in that and the dilemma, for that represented my mother's worst nightmare, this loss of freedom and independence. Yet she knew that there was no other choice, not consistent with her lifelong devotion to her children and her fierce refusal to have them watch her fade into dementia and death.

Then, there is that other moral theme of my mother's life, her profound dread of losing her ability to be "on my own," to lose her independence and ability to choose for herself—from when to sleep to what to eat, or whether to do either. The compromise for her meant no middle ground: she wanted, therefore, to quit, to leave, to die. With "my brain" still intact but her ability to think clearly already becoming impaired, it wasn't dying or death that are expressly mentioned so much as her "sentence" to "jail," her "griping" and "whining," her "gloominess," and that it is "a bad deal." Still, when she talks of watching helplessly her own mother's dying, my mother says she "can't think of a worse way to spend" what life she had remaining in that "prison." She was "glad," she once told a nurse, that "my boys won't have to sit and watch me die," but at the same time often said how she dreaded that very thing happening. And she wanted desperately to "do somethin' about that."

Thus, what she most wanted was precisely what seemed most impossible, and that dilemma was a killing one. The only way any rescue was at all possible—to undergo a kind of moral transformation, a change in the way she viewed her life and her children and herself—was, it turned out, no longer possible for her. "I just can't get up the effort" to get dressed, much less to transform her life.

The trouble, one of the troubles, of course, with the circumstances my mother had to confront and live with, is that people remain seriously uncomfortable with dying, as we are with grief, mourning, and the rest of an all-too-familiar litany. One response to this sort of trouble I learned from Eric Cassell, a rare kind of physician. For someone in my mother's condition, he once wrote, the process of communication with her must be "based on trust. The patient is being told that it is permissible, indeed necessary, to stop doing something that he has done his whole life—namely, battling for life." And, he continues, any time a patient is being given "the bad news," he must also be told that, whatever happens, the physician will give over as much control as humanly possible to the patient—control, for instance, over decisions, but also that he will be given every help in living with pain, grief, sadness, and the rest. Then, "on questions I cannot answer, such as 'How long will I live?' I am also honest, but I often point out how much of the outcome is within the patient's power." The cruncher, then, is this: having made such promises, "it is absolutely essential that the promise be upheld." As Cassell then notes, finally, "to accept that assurance requires a deep trust of one human for another."[3]

Which would have helped my mother enormously. Would it have also helped my brother? Me? I'm not sure, but I think it would. In any event, although I should have known, and done, better, my mother was pretty much left to figure out things for herself, on her own. Then, that second trip to the ER, it was just too late, for she was already half gone, and fully gone only a day or so after transfer from the ER to the ICU. So, truth be told, that "bad news" should have been told to her much earlier; it wasn't. It was only intimated, as it most often is, by nursing home staff, as by her own physician in the small town where she finally was living.

So, she was left to figure it out for herself, at a time when figuring out was just barely part of what she could actually do, if at all. So what then?

She was found, we were told, with her oxygen prongs out of place and her portable oxygen unit turned off, or nearly so. It had been more than four hours since the night nurse at the home had been by her room to check on how she was doing.

The nurse was reported to have said that she stopped by again because nothing had been heard from my mother. Unusual, I suppose, and we were sometimes told that my mother could be "loud," complaining and whining, at any time, late at night, too, I suppose. Her room was not far from the nursing station, so her complaints could be readily heard.

She had not been heard, then, for quite a while. And she was found, it was said, without oxygen, no longer breathing, but it was unclear how long she had been without air. She couldn't complain, for she was not breathing. You have to have air to do that. She didn't have air. She was just lying there. I imagine her there, arms somewhat akimbo, face turned to her left, cheek on the pillow which was slightly moist; she had drooled, her mouth still slightly sagged. On her back. Room awfully quiet.

All but dead by any stretch.

What had happened?

So the nurse did what nurses do: tried to revive, called the EMS, tried to get her doctor, couldn't reach him. Kept working away with the resuscitation, until, finally, the EMS ambulance arrived and the techs took over, bagging and pumping, pushing and checking, forcing air where she had no longer wanted it to be, doing what she did not want done, off to where she did not want to go.

What had happened?

And now, after all these years—that was 1984, and it is as I write 2002—there is no doubt in my mind about what happened. She turned off her portable oxygen unit, she pulled off the prongs, she took the sleeping tablets she had apparently hoarded, it's not clear how many, then she lay back down, on her back, and let it happen, waited for it to happen. She was so tired, worn out, weary with living, working for every single clutch of breath, gasping and grasping and hurting with every slightest movement, utterly exhausted. "It's a bad deal all 'round," she wept into the recorder, and again. "I'm just not getting anywhere, nowhere, no-where," she said, wheezing and gasping. And returned again to a constant theme: "Can't think of a worse sentence . . . th' in . . . than in a nursing home . . . It's just like bein' in jail, really."

So, my mother took things into her own hands, one last, final, desperate grasp at free choice, refusing, too, to sink ever more deeply into sorrow and bitterness, resentment and guilt, haunted every moment by the ghosts of other times and other places, all embedded in her life, herself, now unrecoverable. And she did it with me and my brother centered in her soul: "I'm glad they don't have to sit and watch me die . . . I think I'll spare my children that . . . not that I have any choice about it . . ."

Bereft of meaningful choice, failed by her body, abandoned in the cracks of the healthcare system, forgotten by friends and left by her sons to a "life that isn't any life, not at all," my mother took the last, tiny threads of control of her life—and left with as much dignity as could be had.

Acknowledgments

The gift to my life and understanding by the many patients, families, physicians, nurses, and others with whom I have worked over the past thirty years, I gratefully acknowledge, even though their identities will remain as secret as the sources of insight they allowed me to dwell within. Their generosity of spirit in helping me understand, perhaps unwittingly, the trials of soul each of them went through as I, fumbling and stumbling, earnest all the while, strove to help them get through those troubled times, I also gratefully acknowledge.

My colleagues at the Center for Clinical and Research Ethics at Vanderbilt University clearly deserve far more recognition than I can give them here. Mark Bliton, who many years ago came to study with me and stayed on as a remarkable and valuable colleague: what can I say, Mark, except to tell you how much you made possible for me, how your constant friendship and keen eye shows through so much of what I've since written. And Stuart Finder, now entrusted as director of our little center, who joined our group shortly before Mark completed his doctoral work and helped both Mark and me immeasurably since: Stu, I can think of no one better, more straight and true, to lead the center in the new millennium. I have been fortunate, my words pale images to tell my gratitude to both of you, for years of amazing intellectual and professional companionship, encouragement, and, yes, even hope for a brighter future there. The "field" of ethics in health care, my friends, will be so much the richer for your being involved as you have been. The Friday morning seminar you started so long ago, and ran with such grace and insight, is a standing symbol for what this "field" ought to become. Thank you for that, and for all those years, those times I sometimes felt alone and wasn't.

I am grateful as well to two physicians—mentors, too, each in his own way— Edmund D. Pellegrino and Eric J. Cassell. Their encouragement and insight have been definitive for several generations of us in the medical humanities; they have surely been for me.

I want also to acknowledge, with sincere gratitude, Vanderbilt University Medical Center, its administration, its various hospitals and clinics, and of course the numerous colleagues I came to know and respect during my twenty-one years there, and from whom I learned so much. They may never fully grasp the dimensions of how what would otherwise have been merely possible became, thanks to them, a reality for me. I was not only permitted, but welcomed, into practically any place of practice and was invariably, and eagerly, helped by them all. I could not be more grateful to each of them for enabling me to grapple openly (at times quite awkwardly) with, and eventually to reach some understanding of, the complex, difficult, troubling, and exciting occasions of health care, education, and research that involve them all at that splendid institution.

I am especially grateful to the many Vanderbilt physicians who welcomed me into their practices and helped me establish and sustain the clinical ethics consultation service. I am especially grateful to Josh Billings, M.D., professor emeritus of medicine; Frank Boehm, M.D., director, Division of Maternal-Fetal Medicine, professor of obstetrics and gynecology; Joseph Bruner, M.D., director, fetal diagnosis and therapy, associate professor of obstetrics and gynecology; Ellen Wright Clayton, professor of pediatrics and professor of law; Joseph Cotton, M.D., professor of pediatrics (neonatology); John Flexner, M.D., professor of medicine (hematology/oncology); Virgil LeQuire, M.D., professor of pathology; Grant Liddle, M.D., chair, Department of Medicine; John Oates, M.D., chair (succeeding Dr. Liddle); John S. Sergent, M.D., professor of medicine; Jayant Shenai, M.D., professor of pediatrics (neonatology); Mildred Stahlman, M.D., professor of pediatrics (neonatology); Richard Stein, M.D., professor of medicine (hematology/oncology); and Charles Stratton, M.D., director, clinical microbiology, associate professor of pathology.

Finally, but by no means mere afterthought, for his many years of strong encouragement and quietly definitive discussions, my gratitude goes to John Chapman, M.D., dean of the School of Medicine. I must as well express my gratitude to Steven Gabbe, M.D., the dean newly appointed just when I retired, for his warmth and understanding, and his eagerness to help me in so many ways. And, to Harry Jacobson, M.D., vice-chancellor for health affairs, whose support and encouragement to me, and to the development of a strong ethics program, have been both timely and deeply appreciated.

I want also to record here my profound appreciation to Jeannie Youngkins and Derenda Hodge, distinguished nurses both, and like so many others of their profession efficient and nurturing in that constant in-between where they help patients and families negotiate needed understanding. I hope you know why I owe so much to you and your constant support.

I want to thank them all of them for allowing me, a philosopher, into their midst, and for helping me conceive and gradually carry out a program for clinical practice by philosophers and others in the humanities and social sciences.

Finally, I must again acknowledge my profound gratitude to June Zaner, my wife, for so many incredible, always exciting years, and my children, Melora Zaner-Godsey and Andrew Zaner—you've all made my life charmed.

Everything I've written, here most especially, owes much to others, but only I can and do take responsibility for it.

Notes

Preface

1. James Agee and Walker Evans, *Let Us Now Praise Famous Men* (New York: Houghton Mifflin, 1969), 11.
2. Richard M. Zaner, "Accidents and Time: The Urge to be Normal," in Zaner, *Troubled Voices: Stories of Ethics and Illness* (Cleveland: Pilgrim Press, 1993), 47–56.
3. Richard M. Zaner, *Ethics and the Clinical Encounter* (Englewood Cliffs, N.J.: Prentice Hall, 1988), 225–42, 267–69.
4. Richard M. Zaner, "Power and Hope in the Clinical Encounter: A Meditation on Vulnerability," *Medicine, Health Care, and Philosophy* 3 (2000): 265–75.
5. Richard M. Zaner, "Encountering the Other," in C. S. Campbell and A. Lustig, eds., *Duties to Others*. Theology and Medicine Series, ed. Earl E. Shelp (Boston: Kluwer Academic, 1994), 17–38.
6. Delivered on April 3, 1997.
7. This is one principal theme of a remarkable novel: Simon Mawrer, *Mendel's Dwarf* (New York: Penguin Books, 1998). "[God] has decided on chance as the way to select one combination of genes from another . . . God allows pure luck to decide whether a mutant child or a normal child shall be born" (238).
8. Roger Rosenblatt, "Dreaming the News," *Time* 149, no. 15 (April 14, 1997): 102.
9. Ronald Blythe, "Introduction," *The Death of Ivan Ilyich* (New York: Bantam Books, 1991), 10.

Chapter 1: Quiet Rooms for Troubled Voices

1. An earlier version of this narrative was The Inaugural Christine Martin Lecture, delivered at the University of Melbourne, Melbourne, Australia, April 3, 1997.
2. I tell the fuller story of this below in chapter 6, "The Cruel Clarity of It All."
3. Barry Lopez, *Crow and Weasel* (San Francisco: North Point Press, 1990), 48.
4. As was brilliantly appreciated by Herbert Spiegelberg, "'Accident of Birth': A Non-Utilitarian Motif in Mill's Philosophy," *Journal of the*

History of Ideas 22 (1961), 475–92. This and others of his essays were collected in Herbert Spiegelberg, *Steppingstones toward an Ethics for Fellow
Existers* (The Hague: Martinus Nijhoff, 1986).

5. Simon Mawrer, *Mendel's Dwarf*, 197–98.

6. Mawrer, 238.

7. Roger Rosenblatt, "Dreaming the News," *Time* 149, no. 15 (April 14,
1997): 102.

Chapter 2: When You're Dead, What's to Live For?

1. An earlier version of this reflection appeared as "Illness and the Other,"
in Gerald McKenny and Jonathan R. Sande, eds., *Theological Analyses of
the Clinical Encounter* (Boston: Kluwer Academic, 1994), 185-202. An
earlier version of the story appeared in my book, *Troubled Voices: Stories
of Ethics and Illness* (Cleveland: Pilgrim Press, 1993), chap. 5, "Accidents
and Time: The Urge to Be Normal," 47–56.

2. See, for instance, L. D. Kliever, ed., *Dax's Case: Essays in Medical Ethics
and Human Meaning* (Dallas: Southern Methodist University Press,
1989).

Chapter 3: Hope against Hope

1. An earlier version of this narrative and reflection appeared as "Encountering the Other," in Courtney S. Campbell and B. Andrew Lustig, eds.,
Duties to Others (Boston: Kluwer Academic, 1994), 17–38. In addition, an
earlier and shortened version of the story appeared in my book *Troubled
Voices: Stories of Ethics and Illness* (Cleveland: Pilgrim Press, 1993), chap.
3, pp. 25–36.

2. See Alfred Schutz, *Collected Papers: Studies in Social Theory* (The Hague:
Martinus Nijhoff, 1964) 161, 173; Alfred Schutz and Thomas Luckmann, *The Structures of the Life-World* (Evanston, Ill.: Northwestern
University Press, 1973), 67–98; see also Richard M. Zaner, *The Context
of Self* (Athens: Ohio University Press, 1981), 227–41.

3. See Max Scheler, *The Nature of Sympathy* (New Haven, Conn.: Yale University Press, 1954), 234–51.

4. For a detailed explication of this, see my *Ethics and the Clinical Encounter*
(Englewood Cliffs, N.J.: Prentice Hall, 1988).

5. See Richard M. Zaner, "The Phenomenon of Trust in the Patient-
Physician Relationship," in E. D. Pellegrino, ed., *Ethics, Trust, and the
Professions: Philosophical and Cultural Aspects* (Washington, D.C.: George-
town University Press, 1991), 45–67.

6. Ludwig Edelstein, *Ancient Medicine* (Baltimore: Johns Hopkins University Press, 1967), 329. My reading of the Hippocratic tradition is deeply indebted to the seminal work of this great medical historian.

7. Hans Jonas, "Toward an Ontological Grounding of an Ethics for the Future," in Hans Jonas, *Mortality and Morality: A Search for the Good after Auschwitz*, ed. Lawrence Vogel (Evanston, Ill.: Northwestern University Press, 1996), 101–3.

8. As he emphasized in many places. See my *Ethics and the Clinical Encounter*, chap. 11.

9. Herbert Spiegelberg, "Ethics for Fellows in the Fate of Existence," in Herbert Spiegelberg, *Steppingstones toward an Ethics for Fellow Existers* (The Hague: Martinus Nijhoff, 1986), 199–218.

10. Hans Jonas, *The Imperative of Responsibility: In Search of an Ethics for the Technological Age* (Chicago: University of Chicago Press, 1984), 25–50, 79–109.

11. Herbert Spiegelberg, "Good Fortune Obligates: Albert Schweitzer's Second Ethical Principle," *Ethics* 85 (1975): 232.

12. Alfred Schutz and Thomas Luckmann, *Structures of the Life-World* (Evanston, Ill.: Northwestern University Press, 1973), 86–225.

13. Alfred Schutz, "The Stranger: An Essay in Social Psychology," in Schutz, *Collected Papers II: Studies in Social Theory* (The Hague: Martinus Nijhoff, 1964).

14. This is an interesting instance of the kind of violation mentioned earlier: clearly, although ultimately recognized as a "misunderstanding," Mr. Oland experienced and reacted to Dr. Langston's talk as coercive.

Chapter 4: Don't Let Me Forget to Remember

1. It occurred in spring 1995.

2. The most interesting discussion was with the section of surgery, for whose "grand rounds" I presented an early version of this narrative.

3. Joseph M. Foley, "The Experience of Being Demented," in Robert H. Binstock, Stephen G. Post, and Peter J. Whitehouse, eds., *Dementia and Aging: Ethics, Values, and Policy Choices* (Baltimore: Johns Hopkins University Press, 1992), 30.

4. Eric J. Cassell, "The Nature of Suffering and the Goals of Medicine," *New England Journal of Medicine* 306, no. 11 (March 18, 1982): 639–45.

5. Cited in David H. Smith, "Seeing and Knowing Dementia," in Binstock et al., eds., *Dementia and Aging*, 51.

6. Ibid., 47.

7. Foley, "The Experience of Being Demented," 30.

8. Ibid., 36.

9. Ibid., 37.

10. José Ortega y Gasset, *Man and People* (New York: W. W. Norton, 1957), 18–19, 39–50. As Ortega notes, the word for this exists only in Spanish: *ensimismarse,* "to be inside himself."

11. Smith, "Seeing and Knowing Dementia," 48.

12. Richard J. Martin and Stephen G. Post, "Human Dignity, Dementia, and the Moral Basis of Care Giving," in Binstock et al., eds., *Dementia and Aging,* 58.

13. Smith, "Seeing and Knowing Dementia," 52.

14. Herbert Spiegelberg, *Steppingstones toward an Ethics for Fellow Existers* (The Hague: Martinus Nijhoff, 1986), esp. two essays: "Ethics for Fellows in the Fate of Existence," 199–218; and "Good Fortune Obligates: Albert Schweitzer's Second Ethical Principle," 219–30.

Chapter 5: Broader's Hill

1. Although this story is based on a situation in which I was asked to provide ethics consultation, neither the names, places, nor other identifying characteristics are included. Instead, the events, persons, and circumstances are my own imaginative invention.

Chapter 6: The Cruel Clarity of It All

1. My title for this narrative, plainly, relies on James Agee and Walker Evans, *Let Us Now Praise Famous Men* (New York: Houghton Mifflin, 1969). That work is a constant reminder to me in these stories and ruminations.

2. See my *Ethics and the Clinical Encounter* (Englewood Cliffs, N.J.: Prentice Hall, 1988), 225–42, 267–69.

3. See Eric Cassell, *The Healer's Art: A New Approach to the Doctor-Patient Relationship* (Philadelphia: Lippincott, 1976; reprinted Cambridge, Mass.: MIT Press, 1985), 222–23.